Sauna Detoxification Therapy

To all who have suffered a loss
of family connection because of
the devastating isolation of multiple chemical sensitivities

and especially to my three daughters,
Sacha, *Erin*, and *Alyssa*
who have been the secondary victims
of this modern scourge.

Sauna Detoxification Therapy

A Guide for the Chemically Sensitive

by MARILYN MCVICKER

with a foreword by Richard E. Layton, M.D.
and an introduction by Lawrence A. Plumlee, M.D.

McFarland & Company, Inc., Publishers
Jefferson, North Carolina, and London

This book is not to be construed as medical advice. The ideas and procedures discussed in this book are not intended as substitutes for the medical advice of a trained health professional. The listing of specific products or methods does not constitute an endorsement of those products or methods.

Because multiple chemical sensitivities varies considerably among individuals, it is each person's responsibility to make their own choices based upon personal research, testing of all materials, and professional medical advice. All matters regarding your health require medical supervision. Consult your physician before beginning any program of exercise or sauna detoxification, and before incorporating any ideas discussed in this book. The author and publishers of this book disclaim any liability arising directly or indirectly from the research and ideas presented in this book. —M.M.

This book is printed using soy-based inks on totally chlorine-free paper (except the cover)

British Library Cataloguing-in-Publication data are available

Library of Congress Cataloguing-in-Publication Data

McVicker, Marilyn, 1952–
    Sauna detoxification therapy : a guide for the chemically
sensitive / by Marilyn McVicker ; with a foreword by Richard E.
Layton, and an introduction by Lawrence A. Plumlee.
      p. cm
    Includes bibliographical references and index.
    ISBN 0-7864-0359-4 (sewn softcover : 50# totally chlorine-free paper)
    1. Sauna—Therapeutic use.   2. Chemicals—Health aspects.
3. Allergy—Treatment.   4. Toxicology.   I. Title.
[DNLM: 1. Multiple Chemical Sensitivity—therapy—popular works.
2. Baths, Finnish—popular works.   WD 300 M478s 1997]
RM820.M39   1997
615.8'53—dc21
DNLM/DLC
for Library of Congress   96-51802
                                           CIP

Manufactured in the United States of America

McFarland & Company, Inc., Publishers
  Box 611, Jefferson, North Carolina 28640

Table of Contents

3. Understanding Detoxification

4. Getting Ready

5. Deciding: The Options

List of Figures

Acknowledgments

I would like to thank all the individuals who assisted me in the preparation of this manuscript. Linda Patton spent hours putting the manuscript on disc, logging in additions and corrections, keeping up with a seeming endless stream of work. From the very early stages of the manuscript, Ellen Kinnear donated her support by listening, encouraging, offering cups of tea, and later by donating her editing skills. Evelyn and Vernon Kinnear provided shuttle service to and from the post office and copy store.

I would like to thank my personal physician, Joseph W. Zebley, III, M.D., for his continued support of my primary care. Because he knew me before my chemical injury, he believed the validity of my complaints and rallied to protect me from further injury. He has been supportive as I have weaved my way through the maze of paperwork associated with life as a person with a controversial medical condition.

I want to thank my allergist, Richard E. Layton, M.D., for his invaluable experience with chemical illnesses. He has offered suggestions for many of my complaints, and been creative in tailoring the treatment to my individual needs. Despite major setbacks, he has been unflagging in his support, with excellent and attentive medical care, listening, and encouragement. I also want to thank Dr. Layton for his contribution of a foreword to this book.

Lawrence A. Plumlee, M.D., the president of our local Baltimore Chemical Sensitivities Disorders Association, has become a dear friend during the time we have spent discussing the manuscript. I want to thank him for his suggestions and for also contributing the introduction.

William Drier's illustrations are of the highest calibre. I hold a deep appreciation for his patience in listening to the concepts I wanted and for his willingness to return to his drawing board again and again.

I want to thank the countless individuals from all across the country, too many to mention by name, who so generously took the time to relate to me their experiences with sauna detoxification, sauna purchase, and the design and construction of saunas. I have changed their names to protect their privacy. Special thanks go, however, to Mary Oetzel, Bob Morgan, Carolyn Gorman and Ed Hogan for their kind telephone contributions of experience and expertise.

Cindy Duehring, of Environmental Access Research Network, downloaded information for me from MEDLINE. Cynthia Wilson, editor of *Our Toxic Times,* has provided valuable reprints and up-to-date information and has offered her networking skills and valuable opinions. I want to thank her for introducing me to McFarland.

I would like to thank all the companies listed in the text whose products are less toxic, and who work creatively and sensitively with those of us who need special considerations. I have attempted to list each product with its trademark status. In my work with the marketing and communications departments of these product manufacturers, I was impressed time and again with their willingness to inform, assist and make their products safe for their consumers. I appreciate their cooperation, clarification, and suggestions.

Any products I have suggested are intended only to be included on a personal list of choices. Each product must undergo scrutiny for personal sensitivities or intolerances. No product has been recommended above any other. I apologize for any omission of other appropriate products; the market is changing on a daily basis.

I would also like to thank all those who have provided and funded the research now available on sauna detoxification. Though, undoubtedly, more research is necessary, these physicians, scientists and foundations have accomplished much in the way of important research and documentation.

Finally, I would like to thank my own parents for their part in my tenacious curiosity, drive and determination, and their continued encouragement, support and love.

Marilyn McVicker
November 1996

Foreword

by Richard E. Layton, M.D.

Even though my medical career spans over thirty years, it is only for the past eight that I have become aware of the magnitude of multiple chemical sensitivity. It is now obvious that there has been a startling increase in the number of children who have developed increased recurrent infections, behavioral problems, and developmental delays. In addition, more and more children and adults have developed multiple medical complaints, especially involving the central nervous system, which in my opinion have been caused by a dysregulated immune system. Many of these individuals are also chemically sensitive.

Why is this happening? It is my opinion that over time the air we breathe, the water we drink, and the food we eat have been subjected to more and more pollutants and chemicals. Specifically, pesticides, petroleum products, formaldehyde, perfume, cigarette smoke, and countless other chemicals have caused a dangerous level of pollution that sadly is growing day by day.

Physicians in this country have been well trained in medical school in the science of medicine and are better able to deal with medical problems that can be objectively diagnosed and treated. Physicians usually excel at treating symptoms with medications and surgery. Consequently, in far too many instances, subjective complaints that often occur in the multiple chemical sensitivity (MCS) patient remain unproven by physical exam, laboratory and x-ray findings. These individuals are routinely considered to have psychosomatic illness because of a lack of objectivity in proving the diagnosis. What is obvious to me is not so to a majority of physicians. That is, many patients with MCS do have a significant physical disorder aggravated by the secondary stress of feeling poorly.

Marilyn McVicker's book on sauna detoxification is an excellent resource for coping with the MCS problem. I have already found this

1

work in manuscript form to be very helpful for individuals suffering from multiple chemical sensitivity. With sauna detoxification, the toxic chemicals that are stored in the fatty tissues are released, helping the individual's immune system to re-regulate itself.

Marilyn McVicker has written an excellent text that, if followed, will help many individuals implement a very effective approach for improving health. Ms. McVicker has presented this important information in a concise and understandable way.

I would highly recommend this book to anyone suffering from multiple chemical sensitivity.

Richard E. Layton, M.D.
Specialized Pediatrics, Allergy
and Preventive Medicine
July 1996

Preface

Since 1973 I have been immersed in finding safe therapeutic modalities to facilitate what has become a life-long journey to reclaim the health and quality of life I lost due to multiple and extensive chemical exposures.

For the first part of my illness, I was a working mother. I was experiencing unusual and unexplained health problems. I sought advice from a myriad of doctors and specialists. Despite all the medical advice I was receiving, my condition worsened. Gradually my doctors began to see the relationship between my chemical exposures at work, and my barrage of physical symptoms.

I began to suffer serious reactions to a large array of chemicals and irritants. Eventually, I was confined to bed and could not carry out the tasks associated with daily living; I was unable to care for myself or my children. I became totally disabled and unable to work.

My serious physical symptoms were now compounded by the grief I was experiencing from the loss of my children, my profession, my financial security and my entire way of life. As my physical condition continued to deteriorate, it became apparent that I needed to relocate away from the congestion and pollution of the city.

I was able to locate safe housing outside the city. Over a period of years I slowly emerged from the fog of grief and pain. As my condition improved I was able to search for ways to continue to improve my health. Between the periods of health and relapse, I researched and networked. It became clear that my first step needed to be detoxifying every aspect of my environment.

I removed bottles and cans of common household products. Furniture containing formaldehyde-laden plywood was removed from my living space. I cleaned closets and cupboards; I examined every room, drawer and item. I tested endless bottles of safe soap and shampoo. I implemented nontoxic methods to run my house and complete daily chores.

Through my research I learned of the success of sauna detoxification therapy. I discussed the possibility of this with my environmental health physician. She felt I was too ill and fragile to attempt to travel to a detox center, and advised that I purchase a sauna for home use.

 In 1991, saunas were not yet being advertised in journals for the chemically sensitive. After many calls, I located a manufacturer who promised a nontoxic sauna, free of formaldehyde or glue. I was convinced. I read the sales brochure and sent in my money.

The sauna that arrived was beautiful. However, within 24 hours of being unloaded into the basement I began to develop fevers and other symptoms. The sauna was assembled in the basement, with all windows and doors left open for ample ventilation. I continued to get sicker. How could this be?

My environmental health physician advised that a piece of insulation be sent for laboratory analysis. The report stated that the insulation contained urea formaldehyde foam. I had the sauna totally disassembled and removed to storage. Upon closer examination the carpenter found additional problems with the sauna: hidden pieces of plywood, vinyl coated wood, and even glue.

Once the sauna was removed from the house, I began to improve. In the process, however, I had become more sensitive to products containing formaldehyde. I filed a suit for negligence, negligent misrepresentation and fraud. A long legal battle ensued during which the manufacturer and salesman filed for bankruptcy. I was unable to recover any of my losses.

A friend with multiple chemical sensitivity, aware of my previous experience with saunas, asked me to assist her in developing plans for a custom-made sauna. In exchange for use of her completed sauna, I volunteered to help. I called the major detoxification centers and spoke with the directors. I contacted sauna manufacturers who advertised in magazines and journals geared specifically to the chemically sensitive. I talked with MCS people all across the country, and listened to their experiences with sauna detoxification. I tested lumber and various types of insulation. I researched heaters, hardware, fans and ventilating principles.

The end product of this exhaustive research was a custom-made organic poplar sauna, with a sophisticated filtration and ventilation system. With the use of this sauna, I have continued to improve. I am still disabled with MCS but the improvement in my mental and physical functioning has been significant. I have incorporated sauna therapy into my treatment plan, and have implemented it in a variety of ways. My own individual sauna detoxification program has progressed from weekly saunas to an intense home based detoxification program, and continues with maintenance saunas. My medical care is meticulously monitored by my allergist and my general practitioner, and by regular laboratory analysis of specimens obtained at home. I have continued to focus on the continual detoxification of my total environment: air, food, water, clothing, and even visitors.

As I continued my own program, word spread quickly of my investigation into saunas, and my design of a safe home unit. I began receiving telephone inquiries from other MCS people on a similar search. I heard stories of confusion and clarity, of success and failure. Out of these many conversations came the realization of the need for a book of this type. I began to document my research.

Today, there are many types of safe saunas on the market. Detoxification centers are springing up all across the country. A wide variety of opportunities and alternatives exist. New companies are opening and new products are being developed continually as MCS increases in the population and public awareness.

This book is a guide to asking the right questions. This book is a reference for the consumer in exploring many possibilities for sauna detoxification therapy. I offer it with the hope that others will be able to utilize this information on their own journeys toward improved health.

Marilyn McVicker
November 1996

Introduction

by Lawrence A. Plumlee, M.D.

One of the most surprising aspects of toxic chemical exposure has been the persistence of many chemical and food intolerances at low levels of exposure. Also surprising is that not all exposed persons develop these intolerances. Many of these cases have slowly improved with a reduction of chemical exposure. It seems logical to explore whether improvement could be enhanced by efforts to expel chemical residues from the body. Sauna is one procedure for doing this. Several scientific studies have measured blood and fat samples, patient symptom check lists, and levels of inflammation before and after participation in sauna detoxification programs. The results, to date, are encouraging.

After graduating from Princeton and the Johns Hopkins medical school, and following my internship in internal medicine and post-doctoral fellowship in physiology at Hopkins, I conducted research in psychophysiology at Walter Reed Army Institute of Research. Because of my longstanding interest in public health, I accepted a position as Medical Science Advisor for the research office of the U.S. Environmental Protection Agency. In this position, I was given an opportunity to put scientific information to use for the benefit of the public. My concerns at EPA were the epidemiology and toxicology of low level pollution, not just the effects of acute poisoning. We evaluated chronic everyday exposures to chemicals in society and the workplace. I also learned about such treatments as the use of oral cholestyramine resin to reduce reabsorption of PBBs in workers exposed at Hopewell, Virginia.

In 1976 I met Theron Randolph, M.D., at a meeting of the New York Academy of Sciences. During a banquet, I mentioned my reactivity to garlic to the woman sitting next to me. Dr. Randolph overheard this conversation and offered that he shared a similar reactivity. A conversation ensued and culminated with an invitation for me to come to Chicago and accompany him on his rounds. In 1977 I took him up on his offer. I was utterly astounded as I spoke to one patient after another reporting illness of unknown etiology: chronic arthritis, chronic colitis, chronic enteritis, multiple sclerosis, mental and emotional problems, lupus, chronic skin and respiratory problems including asthma. After entering his environmentally clean medical unit, the patients fasted on water alone for four or five days, and usually found a remarkable clearing of their symptoms for the first time in many years. From almost every patient I heard similar results. Following this initial fasting period, organic foods were then introduced, one at a time, until each patient had a number of foods that could be safely eaten without adverse effects. Dr. Randolph then introduced a commercially grown, prepared, canned variety of the tolerated food. Many patients were not able to tolerate food grown, processed and packaged with the use of chemicals, pesticides and other synthetic additives. Dr. Randolph took this opportunity to advise his patients about chemically less-contaminated living, and sent them home to continue the process of sorting out their food and environmental intolerances.

It was an amazing experience to witness a variety of illnesses of unknown etiology provoked or controlled by the presence or absence of ordinary foods and chemicals. To witness Dr. Randolph's reasonable approach to dealing with food and chemical reactivities was heartening to me. I was seeing common illnesses that were being provoked by everyday foods and chemicals. I was seeing the same people clear completely of these illnesses and brought into remission by avoiding the same common foods and chemicals. Naturally, I was enthusiastic about bringing this to the attention of my colleagues at the EPA, NIH, FDA, OSHA, NIOSH, the Consumer Product Safety Commission and the Centers for Disease Control. I was eager to have other scientists and medical personnel investigate Dr. Randolph's observations. I wanted to interest them in facilitating additional research.

In 1977 while attending a meeting of the Society for Clinical Ecology, I had the opportunity to meet other physicians who were validating Dr. Randolph's findings in their own practices. I continued my own personal observations by visiting William Rea, M.D., in Dallas, Texas and accompanying him on his daily rounds through his own clean ward. Again, I saw patients experiencing symptoms from low level chemical and food exposures.

In 1983 I traveled to San Diego to speak at a meeting of chemically sensitive patients. During this trip I first saw that physicians were advocating sauna detox at the local Health Med program in the Los Angeles area, and were introducing similar programs in their private practices as a treatment for multiple food and chemical sensitivities. This was the first I had heard of sauna being used for this purpose. Subsequently Dr. Rea and others offered this treatment.

Dr. Randolph, who first described multiple food and chemical sensitivities in the 1950s, calling them "ecological illnesses," theorized that the temporary worsening of fasting patients was due to withdrawal from addictive substances. I wondered if the increase of symptoms was due to mobilization of chemicals from the fat where they were stored. Hearing Dr. Rea's enthusiasm, Dr. Randolph sent some of his patients for sauna detoxification. In the late 1980s, he enthusiastically reported at the annual International Symposium on Man's Health and the Environment that he was finding some patients who were improving after sauna detox, after not responding to mere avoidance of chemical incitants. He reported the successful use of sauna as sometimes crucial and effective in reducing chemical sensitivities even when long term environmental and dietary controls had failed.

There is a need for more research data indicating that environmental exposures are associated with and are the cause of multiple food and chemical sensitivities. If one can show that residues of chemicals are reduced by sauna, and that there is simultaneously a clinical recovery and improvement, then this adds evidence to support the theory that chemical exposures can cause multiple chemical and food sensitivities. If you can enhance the metabolism of toxic chemicals from the body such that they are removed more rapidly or detoxified to a less-toxic metabolic breakdown product, i.e., broken down to less toxic chemicals within the body, and clinical improvement follows, there is opportunity for scientific advancement. It is extremely important for society to know that commonly occurring chemicals are causing disease at commonly encountered levels. More importantly, it often provides relief for the victims of illness from chemical poisoning.

Another method of removing toxic chemical residues from the body is the use of food supplements to restore detoxification metabolism. Biochemists have long known that metabolic enzymes can be activated by increasing the nutrients which generate them or assist them, and by removing the end-products of the metabolism. It has been decades since William Philpott, M.D., and H.L. Newbold, M.D., began using food supplements for multiple chemical sensitivities. Recent scientific analyses of the detoxification pathways by Jeffrey Bland, Ph.D., and others, have led to the development of better rationales for supplements, which apparently help restore and enhance the body's normal methods for clearing toxic substances from the tissues with a minimum of damage. These dietary supplements are expected to enhance sauna detoxification and do more than replace minerals sweated out of the body. For example, several supplements in the category of antioxidants have been proven to reduce the toxic damage of ingested chemicals. In addition, these antioxidants are expected to reduce tissue damage when toxic chemicals which have been stored in the fat, are mobilized by sauna and re-enter the bloodstream. Scientific examination of these hypotheses should be a high research priority.

We do not know why some patients get worse for long periods after sauna. It is thought to be due to toxic damage from remobilized chemicals. Perhaps enzyme systems are poisoned instead of improved by increased toxins in the blood. Hans Selye and others observed that the same stressor which heightened physical performance could lead to illness if the stresses were prolonged or excessive. Users of the sauna would do well to remember this. Wise patients do not rely solely on their doctors, but also monitor their own symptoms to challenge their bodies without incurring excessive stress. Experience is often the best teacher. Meanwhile, scientific efforts are needed to determine who is most likely to benefit and who will not, and to lay out the optimal conditions for success.

It is lamentable that more effort has not been placed on research devoted to detoxification. The scientific community has been too wary of the protestations of the chemical industry, which maintains that the absence of a consistent mechanism to explain multiple food and chemical reactivity argues against the biological origins of the phenomenon. As a result, patients have suffered from the scarcity of viable treatment options which have been proven effective. The time has come to explore and document how the proven chemical residues in patients' bodies may be lowered in ways that reduce patient complaints.

The use of sauna and hot baths has been used as a healing modality for thousands of years. In this country, the American Indians used sweat lodges for healing. The Spanish Conquistadores also found native Americans using hot water bathing for healing. Hot Springs, Arkansas, is the oldest national park, hosting a spa predating the Spanish, who "discovered" it in the 1500s. Sauna detoxification is not a new phenomenon, but an ancient healing modality being used to assist in current medical situations.

In this book, Marilyn McVicker pulls no punches, but realistically portrays the successes and the failures, the precautions and the difficulties that some patients encounter. The book is intended to help readers decide upon their own participation in a program of sauna detoxification. She arms her readers with scientific documentation supporting the medical validity of sauna detoxification in reducing chemicals stored in fat tissues, as well as in reducing patient symptoms and complaints. The information offered in the second chapter of her book will be a valuable tool to patients attempting to inform their physicians, health insurance carriers, and employers. This book educates the readers to advocate for themselves by exploring many of the facets of this method of treatment.

> *Lawrence A. Plumlee, M.D.*
> October 1996

1. The Issue
of Chemical Illness

Our Toxic World

There is an increasing percentage of the population which is suffering from exposures to the toxic chemicals surrounding us. The sufferings of this population range from mild to severe and life-threatening. Chemicals surround us, not only in the air we breathe, but in virtually every aspect of our lives, our food, water, medicine, clothing and cosmetics.

News media broadcasts frequently include coverage of chemical spills, diseased fish in polluted waters, lowered air quality standards, and burning oil wells. We are bombarded with reports of immune system diseases, misunderstood disorders, and untreatable maladies. We hear stories about sick buildings, about workers who became ill following chemical exposures. We hear of children born to mothers who ingested chemical prescriptions, and families developing cancer from drinking contaminated water, eating contaminated meat, or living near hazardous waste sites.

Current literature includes personal accounts disclosing the catastrophes of veterans exposed to Agent Orange, of Michigan farmers and residents contaminated by deadly polybrominated biphenyls (PBBs). We hear news reports about asbestos workers, children ingesting lead paint, the dangers of dioxin, DDT, carbon monoxide, sulfur dioxide, passive cigarette smoke, and silicone breast implants.

The Environmental Protection Agency (EPA) and the National Institute for Occupational Safety and Health (NIOSH) have passed laws to set standards concerning pollution and toxic substances. Even

13

though "safe levels" of various chemicals have been proposed, no one really knows exactly what levels are safe, or for that matter, what levels are dangerous.

Many physicians feel that the existing limits on chemical exposures are misleading. In fact, many illness reactions occur following repeated "low level" chemical exposures.[1]* The guidelines set by the EPA as "safe," may, in fact, not be "safe" at all. What may be safe for one person may be extremely dangerous for another.

According to the National Research Council, toxicity data are not available for 80 percent of the 49,000 chemicals in daily use.[2] Of the chemicals for which we *do* have toxicity data, the data are useless in establishing guidelines for exposure limits. The knowledge that certain substances are definitively toxic far exceeds the regulations and standards set to protect the public.

It is a fact that exposure to toxic contaminants and hazardous chemicals can precipitate or contribute to a variety of illnesses in an exposed population.

Illness and Toxicity

It is estimated that 15 percent of the population has become sensitized to common household and commercial chemicals. For some people, this is a minor problem. For others, it may be serious and disabling. Reactions to chemicals can be immediate or delayed, mild or life threatening.

Multiple chemical sensitivities, or MCS, is a disease or disorder caused by exposure to chemicals. Chemicals contained in food, air, clothing, and personal products can trigger an array of physical, emotional, neurological and psychological symptoms. The onset of MCS may be sudden or gradual. Other names for this type of illness include environmental illness, ecological illness, E.I., chemical hypersensitivity syndrome, total allergy syndrome, and 20th century disease.

An individual may experience the symptoms of multiple chemical sensitivities following one massive exposure to a toxic chemical, or following repeated low level exposures. Some individuals can pinpoint the

*References are found beginning on page 149.

specific exposure which caused the beginning of their symptoms. Other individuals cannot remember any event which may have triggered their conditions.

Many factors weigh in determining an individual's susceptibility to developing MCS: the amount and strength of the chemical, the length of the exposure, a person's genetic, physical and emotional health, age, sex, and previous exposures; all these factors work together in determining the degree of susceptibility to chemically related illness. Certain populations seem to be more susceptible than others. They include women, children, the elderly, unborn children, those people already suffering from allergies or immune system dysfunctions, and those people who are exposed to chemical incitants in their work place. Populations at greater risk of suffering an accidental exposure to toxic chemicals would include those individuals working in buildings with poor air quality, those living near landfills or toxic waste dumps, individuals living or working in areas of severe pollution, and industrial workers. In addition, chemicals are known to exacerbate the symptoms of many chronic illnesses and autoimmune disorders.

There are two reasons which may explain why one person is able to tolerate an environmental exposure and another may not. First, the total load or total body burden is the total amount of chemical contaminants, bacteria, and viruses which strain the individual's detoxification metabolism. This concept has been likened to a barrel, or row boat, which when full begins to sink. The greater an individual's total body burden, the greater the possibility of an illness reaction.

The second reason for individual responses to environmental contaminants, is the ability of the body to adapt to particular chemicals or environments. Often an individual may not notice the toxic effects of a particular situation because their body has the ability to temporarily tolerate the toxicity, and mask the symptoms of the exposure. This phenomenon, known as masking, often plays a part in the inability of certain persons to connect various exposure situations with illness responses. The harmful effects of the chemical exposure may develop many months or years later, as the total load or total body burden of the individual increases.

The symptoms and complaints of an individual presenting with multiple chemical sensitivities cover a wide range of possibilities. These symptoms may seem unusual and unrelated, and are often discounted as emotional or hysterical reactions. Sometimes the onset of MCS can cause symptoms which are delayed or localized, and which may appear to be an "allergy." As time progresses and more chemicals become absorbed by the body, reactions may become more severe and systemic, and develop into a chronic condition involving more organ systems of the body. These serious reactions can often be triggered by diminishing amounts of offensive chemicals. In addition, it is notable that many individuals become sensitive to a larger number of chemicals and experience an increasing diversity of symptoms. This phenomenon is known as "spreading."[3]

Symptoms of multiple chemical sensitivities include:

Central Nervous System

Tiredness	Headaches	Inadequate reading
Exhaustion	Confusion	comprehension
Depression	Memory loss	Difficulty with word
Nervousness	Hyperactivity	retrieval
Weakness	Dizziness	Inadequate verbal
Irritability	Tremors	comprehension
Insomnia	Seizure disorders	
Tension	Anxiety	

Gastrointestinal System

Dryness	Bloating	Colitis
Increased salivation	Constipation	Gall bladder pain
Canker sores	Diarrhea	Hunger
Nausea	Gas	Cramps

Musculoskeletal System

Joint pain	Muscle spasms	Stiffness
General edema	Weakness	
Arthritis	Wasting	

Cardiovascular System

Rapid heartbeat	Skipped beats	Tingling
Irregular heartbeat	Chest pain	Circulation problems

Left arm pain
Nosebleed
Hypertension
Migraines

Vasculitis
Faintness
Spontaneous bruising
Phlebitis

Hot flashes
Raynaud's disease
Myocardial infarcts

Respiratory System

Shortness of breath
Asthma
Wheezing

Frequent colds
Bronchitis
Tight chest

Reactive airways
Cough

Eye, Ear, Nose and Throat

Nasal congestion
Sneezing
Nasal itching
Runny nose
Postnasal drip
Sore throat
Dry throat
Cough

Hoarseness
Earaches
Itching ears
Hearing loss
Vertigo
Imbalance
Watery eyes
Itching eyes

Dry eyes
Blurring
Double vision
Pain in eyes
Loss of vision
Twitching eyelids
Swollen eyelids
Irritated eyes

Skin

Itching
Flushing
Burning
Hot or cold

Tingling
Excessive sweat
Rashes
Hives

Blotches
Red spots
Acne
Eczema

Genitourinary System

Frequent urination
Painful urination
Loss of bladder

control
Vaginal discharge
Vaginal itching

Vaginal irritation or
   swelling

The Response of the Medical Community

The response of the medical community to MCS makes the diagnosis and treatment of this disease difficult. Patients are often disbelieved, told their symptoms are psychosomatic, and discounted. There are a limited number of physicians with training and experience in environmental and chemical illness. The average family physician has received fewer than four hours of training in nutrition, toxicology, and occupational medicine. As a result, many patients circulate from specialist to specialist accumulating a variety of diagnoses and pharmaceuticals, and little in the way of relief from their symptoms. Many patients are often misdiagnosed or not diagnosed at all. A definitive diagnosis of MCS is often difficult to obtain.

There is great controversy in the medical community over the existence of MCS. Patients suffering from chemical exposures are often caught in the crossfire between family physicians, traditional allergists, occupational physicians, ear, nose and throat specialists, and the opinions of other specialists they may have sought for professional assistance. To add to this stress, MCS patients are often embroiled in the quagmire of the legal arena as they seek to obtain financial remuneration for their injuries. Even when a patient is fortunate to find a physician who is supportive, patients are often confused by the lack of agreement on a clear definition of the disorder by those in the field.

The bitter controversy surrounding MCS and its diagnosis and treatment has resulted in an extremely confusing and hazardous journey for the patient. The lack of funding, research and professional agreement have led to different treatment approaches, most of which are experimental. Once a treatment is received, it can be difficult to obtain reimbursement through health insurance plans which do not accept the diagnosis of MCS, or any of the various treatment modalities offered.

Various physicians and specialists continue to pose various explanations and treatments. Some physicians are studying the effects of pesticides, herbicides, Candida, parasites, house dust, and dust mites, on their patients with MCS. Other physicians have proposed connections between MCS and sick building syndrome, Gulf war syndrome, Legionnaires' disease, cacosmia (acute sense of smell that causes illness reactions), mercury amalgam used in dental fillings, and time-dependent sensitization.

Gunnar Heuser, M.D., Ph.D., FACP has completed studies which show an elevation of TA1 (CD26) cells, an increase of chemical antibodies and auto-antibodies, as well as abnormal SPECT (single photon emission computed tomography) scans following an accidental or intentional chemical exposure.[4] William Meggs, M.D., Ph.D., and Crawford

H. Cleveland, Jr., M.D., have noticed an increase of nasal abnormalities and nasal resistance in patients with MCS, suggesting that these patients have an increase in upper-airway disease.[5] Stephen A. Schacker, M.D., has offered the opinion that MCS is a disease where inhalation of chemicals injure the hippocampus and limbic areas of the brain.[6] This explanation, he proposes, accounts for the memory loss, emotional symptoms, and other cognitive impairments that are associated with damage to the limbic lobe of the brain.

Thomas J. Callendar, M.D., is widely known for his research using PET scans and SPECT scans to show that inhalation of chemicals causes a decrease of cerebral blood flow, and a resultant loss of brain function. His studies reveal that the areas of the brain most often affected by chemical injury and resulting toxic encephalopathy are the frontal and temporal lobes, and the basal ganglia.[7]

In addition, physicians are studying the link between MCS and porphyria. In the past porphyria has been considered a rare inherited disorder although there are well documented cases caused by exposure to specific chemicals and drugs. Porphyria involves a deficiency of enzymes that causes an increase in one or several of the porphyrins which become deposited in the tissues and cause illness. There are specific laboratory tests to detect the presence of this disease. William Morton, M.D., William Morton, M.D., Dr. PH, of Oregon Health Sciences University, noticed that some of his patients suffering from toxic exposures shared symptoms similar to porphyria. The testing of his patients led to the discovery of porphyria in a large percentage of patients suffering from MCS.[8]

Practitioners of modern medicine have offered prescription medications and other conventional treatments which have provided little relief, and which have sometimes exacerbated the symptoms of multiple chemical sensitivities. Up to this time, the basic "treatment" for MCS has been strict avoidance of the chemicals and environmental situations which incite reactions.

Physicians who have traditionally treated MCS have been trained in occupational or environmental medicine. Another field of medicine, clinical ecology, was started by Theron Randolph, M.D., in the 1950s. Originally trained in internal medicine, and later receiving his fellowship in allergy and immunology, he named this new field *clinical ecology* as a way of emphasizing its belief in environmental incitants (rather than immunoglobulinE [IgE] mediated allergies) as the causative factor in chemical sensitivities.

In 1990, Stephen R. Barron, M.D., CCFP, conducted a survey of 29 persons with multiple chemical sensitivities for the Canada Mortgage and Housing Corporation. These participants completed detailed questionnaires about their symptoms and treatment. Approximately half of the respondents with MCS sought medical help from six to ten physicians. Of these, the seven most often mentioned were general practitioners, traditional allergists, clinical ecologists, ear, nose and throat specialists, psychiatrists, internists, and neurologists. The respondents also listed alternative practitioners. Among these, the three most often mentioned were chiropractors, naturopaths, and homeopaths.[9]

It is noted that although the respondents initially sought help from traditional sources, they did not find relief from their symptoms. This led the participants to try a variety of alternative treatments. The treatments listed as the most beneficial were the treatment options associated with avoidance of chemicals, i.e., avoidance in living environment, diet, water, air, and general lifestyle choices involving a lower contact with synthetic chemicals.[10]

A 1995 MCS Treatment Evaluation Survey by Leonard A. Jason, Ph.D., of DePaul University listed eight treatments specifically for MCS. These were avoiding allergenic foods, avoiding chemical exposures, creating a "safe place," moving to a cleaner environment, neutralizations to foods, neutralizations to chemicals, sauna detoxification, and air filters.[11]

Other treatment modalities for MCS include the following treatments listed in alphabetical order:

Acidophilus	Desensitization
Acupuncture	DHEA
Allergy injections	Digestive enzymes
Antidepressant medication	Echinacea
Antifungal medication	Enzyme potentiated desensitiza-
Biofeedback	tion (EPD)
B-12 injections	Filtered water
Candida treatment	Gamma globulin
Chinese herbs	Garlic
Chiropractic	Guided imagery
Coffee enemas	Herbal supplements
Colonics	Homeopathy
CoQ10	Hydrogen peroxide therapy

Hypnosis
Juicing
L-Glutathione
Magnesium shots
Massage
Meditation
Mercury amalgam removal
Naturopath
Organic food
Phenolics
Prayer

Prescribed oxygen
Provocation-neutralization
Relaxation techniques
Rest
Rotation diet
Steroids
Support groups
Therapy or counseling
Vitamin C
Vitamins and supplements

It is clear that MCS patients are very ill and in desperate need of medical assistance. Some patients elect to stay within the perceived safety-net of conservative physicians and allergists. Others seek assistance from physicians trained in clinical ecology. Many patients have taken advantage of the alternative therapies available. For the chemically sensitive patient, the choice can be confusing and frightening.

The Need for Early Intervention

Some chemical sensitivity illnesses develop with repeated low-level exposures over a long period of time. Others are triggered by a single toxic exposure. The minor symptoms that accompany the onset of chemical sensitivities often are mistakenly diagnosed as common health problems. It is difficult at this early stage to obtain an accurate diagnosis.

It is at this early point in the onset of chemically related illness that a safe and effective intervention is needed. In a conservative effort to proceed cautiously, many physicians have taken a "wait and see" approach. However, it is at this crucial point in the early stages of the development of chemical-related illnesses that a safe and effective intervention is necessary before the damage becomes impossible to reverse.

Chemicals are often overlooked as a causative agent in these subacute and acute conditions. If the chemical connection is not recognized and eliminated, the patient continues to function within the toxic situation. Unexplored and misdiagnosed, the health problems continue, or increase.

2. Sauna History and Research

History

Sauna ("sow-na" or "saw-na") refers to a dry heat perspiration bath, or the room in which such a bath is taken. Traditionally, bathers sit or lie on wood benches and perspire freely at temperatures from 160° to 212° F. A sauna is taken for the purpose of cleansing and relaxation. The dry heat of a sauna contains less than 30 percent humidity and increases circulation, relaxes muscular tension, and enhances the excretion of wastes. This method of bathing is believed to have a cleansing effect on the body. It is physically and mentally beneficial, as well as a relaxing and invigorating social experience.

Traditionally, an initial sauna is usually followed by a swim, shower, or romp in the snow to cool down. The bather then returns to the hot sauna for another bath. This scenario is usually repeated several times. There are many variations in the type of building, heat source, temperature, length of stay and method of cool-down. The sauna experience is different for everyone, as each sauna is different and each person's reaction to heat varies.

In Finland, this dry-heat form of bathing has been a custom for over two thousand years. Other societies have practiced the art as well. The Greeks, Romans, Russians, Slavs, Turks, Africans, Germans, Eskimos, Irish, Mexicans, Mayans, and North American Indians have all shared a history of some form of perspiration bathing.[12]

In Finland, the sauna is a basic part of life. It is believed that saunas outnumber automobiles. Saunas are commonly owned by homeowners and even offered in apartments and urban dwellings. Saunas are so necessary to the Finnish way of life that they are often built before the house. Saunas are not only used for relaxation and quiet enjoyment, but are an intrinsic part of social life.

Traditionally, Finns set aside one evening a week when family and friends gather. The heater is started with wood. After the sauna is hot (or "ripened") the bathers enter, with children taking the lower cooler seats, and the adults gravitating to the hotter upper benches. After everyone has begun to perspire, the bathers leave the sauna for a cool-down period. This can be a roll in the snow, a swim in a nearby water hole, or any number of invigorating options. Following this, everyone returns to the sauna where water is ladled from a wooden bucket over the hot sauna rocks. This action produces steam and makes the sauna hotter, increasing perspiration. The bathers use bundles of birch twigs tied together to stimulate or whisk their skin, increasing circulation, and assisting the body in continuing to perspire freely. This scenario is repeated several times, until bathers finish with showers, a final invigorating swim, and the sharing of a snack.

It is believed that the Finnish immigrants brought the first sauna to America in the 1600s. Sauna remained a Finnish custom in this country until the 1950s when Americans, initially suspicious of the practice, began to appreciate its benefits. By the 1960s, sauna was widely practiced and began to appear in American homes, resorts, health clubs, and spas.

Sauna has been used for certain physical ailments; for example, to assist in healing from colds, arthritis, congestion, allergies, poor circulation, acne and headaches. Many athletes use sauna in conjunction with massage following strenuous workouts. Sauna is often a part of health centers, and physical therapy programs.

Spas and Hot Tubs

The benefits of hot baths, or hydrotherapy, have been known by doctors for a long time. In the last several years spas and hot tubs have become fashionable. Most people have had the opportunity to enjoy a relaxing bath either in their own home, the home of a friend, or at a hotel, resort, or apartment complex.

Hot baths have a history in many cultures. The Egyptian, Greek and Turkish people have long enjoyed hot water bathing. More notably, the Romans and Japanese have traditions that have led to spas and hot tubs as we know them today. Roman baths were centered around social contact, and were busy centers of activity built to accommodate thousands of bathers at one time. The Japanese *ofuro* was an entirely different experience in that it was a large wooden tub located in a family setting and primarily used by a solitary individual for meditation and relaxation.

In America we have combined the social and meditative qualities of hot water bathing. Mineral hot springs were available in Santa Barbara, California, in the early 1900s. As progress continued, local people began building hot tubs from discarded wine vats, old water tanks, and barrels. By the 1960s the hot springs had moved from the canyons surrounding Santa Barbara to the backyards of local homeowners.

Early commercial spas were built of *gunite*, a tedious and costly process involving sand and cement. Gradually, spa construction has evolved to lighter weight, less expensive materials. Modern spas are fashioned of thermoplastic and acrylic materials, and are less expensive, bringing the ownership of spas well within the reach of more homeowners.

Spas and hot tubs are similar in that they both offer a bathing experience in hot water that is kept at a temperature of 100° to 104°. Hot tubs and spas differ in their construction, maintenance and use.

Hot tubs are usually built of wood, and are beautiful in their rustic simplicity. The look, feel and ambiance of wood creates a warm and meditative experience. Most hot tubs are built of redwood, cedar, teak, or oak. The classic design has been unchanged for years. Because the hot tub is constructed of wood, it must be kept filled with water. If it is allowed to dry out for more than two days, the tub will leak between the staves when the tub is refilled. Water chemistry must be precise to protect the wood and keep down the growth of bacteria. Because of the depth of hot tubs and the porous surface of the wood, draining and scrubbing is more difficult than for spas. A "spa-tub" is a wooden hot tub with a plastic liner. This plastic liner decreases the chance of leaking and allows for easier cleaning.

Spas started out as whirlpool baths, used for medicinal or therapeutic reasons. Because they provided a wonderful experience for the bather, their use became more widespread. Spas are sleek and boxy.

They can be in-ground units built by a contractor and surrounded by a deck and luxurious landscaping, or smaller portable units similar to any other household appliance. Most spas are made with plastic surfaces: acrylic, some of the new ABS (acrylonitrile-butadiene-styrene) plastics, or other similar weatherable polymers. Both the in-ground and portable versions come pre-wired, and are easy to install, and easy to clean.

Both spas and hot tubs are rapidly gaining in popularity as new styles and features become available. A thorough knowledge of water chemistry is important in operating and maintaining both a hot tub and a spa. Good sanitation is vital. Although there are innovative techniques for sanitization using ultraviolet light, hydrogen peroxide, and ozone, it is likely that stronger disinfectants and chemicals will be needed to maintain the tub safely and efficiently. For these reasons hot tubs and spas are not usually recommended for those persons with multiple chemical sensitivities.

Detoxification Baths

Hot water baths increase circulation, and cause perspiration much in a similar fashion to saunas. Hot water causes the pores to open and wastes to excrete through the skin. Capillary action increases and the cardiovascular system works harder as the body excretes toxins through the various organs of detoxification. Many persons with MCS have found success with soaks in a simple home bath of hot water.

As with undertaking any regimen, it is important to talk with your physician. Detoxification baths can cause an exacerbation of symptoms and can be dangerous for certain people. Do not try these on your own without your physician's guidance, and for your safety do not attempt to take them without another person nearby. Stop immediately if you begin to feel sick, exhausted, dizzy, or nauseous, or develop a headache while you are in the bath.

Before taking a detoxification bath make certain you and your tub are clean. Wash it thoroughly before you fill the tub, so that you are not soaking in dirty water. Use only safe, filtered water, that does not contain harmful chemicals. Submerge your entire body up to your neck, so you receive the full benefit of the soak. Be certain to replace your fluids during and after the bath. Extra vitamin and mineral supplementation is essential to replace what you sweat out. Begin slowly, with short baths of five minutes, increasing only as you are able, to a maximum of 30 minutes. If you become too hot, or experience illness symptoms while in the tub, do not attempt to get up out of the tub. Serious injury could result from a fall in a slippery tub. Instead, drain the tub as you are reclining in it, allowing your body to cool down slowly. Exit the tub when the severe symptoms subside. Many people find that several detox baths a week bring a gradual improvement to their health.[13]

Other Methods of Sweating

Other methods of sweating can provide the release of toxins and a beneficial experience. Exercise has been proven to provide unparalleled benefits to the entire body. Exercise programs should be started with the advice and guidance of a physician who is aware of your total health. Some individuals with MCS have exercised in sweat clothing, to help induce and increase the amount of perspiration excreted by the body. Steam baths can be beneficial because they cause sweating, but care should be exercised if the steam bath is contaminated with chemicals used to remove or retard mold growth.

Sauna Research

Toxic chemicals, volatile organic compounds and pesticides can be found in all parts of the body. These chemicals have been stored in the organs, tissues, fatty deposits, brain and nervous system, and are not totally dispelled during the normal processes of elimination.

Lipid tissue is located in organs throughout the body, and has been found to have a particular ability to store toxic chemicals. Lipid tissue comprises what we commonly refer to as "fat," and is the primary component of the neurological system, brain, neurons, and neurotransmitters.

The aim of chemical detoxification is to remove the stores of toxic chemicals from the lipid tissue of the body. There has been a wealth of research proving the validity of sauna detoxification for those injured or contaminated with lipophilic chemicals.

In 1972 Richard D. Swartz, M.D., Swartz, M.D., Captain, Medical Corps, United States Army, and Frederick R. Sidell, M.D., of the Biomedical Laboratory in Edgewood, Maryland, completed a study on the elimination of pralidoxime. Pralidoxime chloride is used in the treatment of organophosphate poisoning. Six healthy enlisted Army personnel volunteered and passed extensive physical examinations. The researchers found that a program of exercise and heat caused a change in the distribution of the drug by changing the pattern of plasma flow, thus affecting the renal elimination and metabolism of the drug.[14]

In the mid–1970s, according to researchers at the Foundation for Advancements in Science and Education (FASE), L. Ron Hubbard was working with previous users of LSD (lysergic acid diethylamide). He realized that sometimes these individuals experienced reactions similar to their initial experience with the drug, only years later and without the use of any drugs at all. Like many other chemicals, LSD is stored in the lipid tissue of the body.

In response to this problem Mr. Hubbard developed a "sweat program" in 1977, and tried it on people who were chronic users of heavy drugs and narcotics. The program was a success. It was evident that in addition to releasing the drugs and narcotics from the system, the program was causing the release of other toxins and stored lipophilic chemicals. L. Ron Hubbard's detoxification program was formally released as the Purification Program in 1979 and was applied to individuals suffering from the effects of many lipophilic drugs and chemicals.[15]

In 1978 James R. Cohn, M.S., and Edward A. Emmett, M.B., B.S., M.S., FRACP, tested the excretion of trace metals in human sweat. Following an exact collection protocol they found that sweat was a vital vehicle for the elimination of zinc and copper. In addition, more nickel and cadmium were found to be excreted in sweat samples than in urine.[16]

Meanwhile, an unfortunate thing was happening in the State of Michigan. The Michigan Chemical Corporation manufactured two products: a magnesium oxide additive for livestock feed, and the flame retardant PBB which was used primarily in plastic production. Polybrominated biphenyl is similar in its toxic effects to its cousin PCB (polychlorinated biphenyl) in that it is considered hepatoxic, neurotoxic, immunotoxic, and carcinogenic. In mid–1973, a batch of PBB was mistaken for the magnesium oxide supplement and accidentally dumped into the livestock feed in central Michigan. Before anyone realized what had happened, the feed was sold and used by farmers all over the state. The dairy cattle began to show signs of contamination: their milk production decreased, they developed abnormal hooves, became lame, and started spontaneously aborting calves. Scores of cattle were sold into the food chain and consumed by human beings in the form of meat, milk, butter, and cheese. Other types of livestock were also contaminated. Farm families began experiencing troubling and nightmarish health consequences, showing impaired liver and immune system functioning, neurological disturbances, and other serious manifestations. Michigan residents who had been eating the contaminated food began experiencing symptoms, as well. By the time the deadly mix-up was discovered, nine million Michigan residents had been poisoned. New studies have shown PBB in the environment and food chain of 13 additional states.[17]

In response to the problem in Michigan, Wolff, Anderson, Rosenman and Selikoff, from the Environmental Sciences Laboratory at Mount Sinai School of Medicine in New York, launched a study calibrating the amount of PBB stored in the blood and fat of Michigan residents. In 1976 they tested 993 Michigan dairy workers and 55 chemical employees and found 96 percent to have concentrations greater than 0.3 parts per billion (ppb). At the same time they tested a control group of Wisconsin dairy farm residents and detected only 5 percent who had levels of PBB above 0.3 ppb. Of this 5 percent of Wisconsin dairy farmers, five out of the eight individuals were persons who had recently moved to Wisconsin from Michigan.

In 1977 these individuals were reexamined. The measurements for serum and adipose PBB were highly consistent with the previous findings. In 1978 individuals were again reexamined, with no outstanding difference in serum levels of PBB. It was notable that several of the chemical workers had increased values, suggesting that perhaps they were continuing to be exposed to the chemical. These findings led researchers to believe that the body burden levels of stored PBB were remaining constant, or that the PBB levels had not decreased since the previous testing.[18]

In 1982, Wolff, Anderson and Selikoff began to study the serum and adipose residues of a statistically larger portion of Michigan residents to determine the contamination levels in various parts of the state. This study measured 1,738 participants, 97 percent of whom showed

PBB residues in their serum or adipose. The highest levels were found in the farm families and those living in areas where the livestock farms were eventually quarantined. The levels of PBB were lowest in areas of the state farthest removed from the contaminated farms. In addition to measuring PBB levels, the testers measured PCB and DDE—2,2'-bis-(p-chlorophenyl)-1,1-dichloroethylene (PIP'-DDE), a dichlorodiphenyl-trichloroethane (DDT) residue—in the serum of various age groups. Their findings suggested that these chemicals were readily in the environment, and accumulated with age.[19]

In 1982 a study was published by the Foundation for Advancements in Science and Education (FASE), under the direction of D.W. Schnare, G. Denk, M. Shields, and S. Brunton. The purpose of the study was to test the validity of a detoxification program which had been developed to assist in the reduction of body stores of recreational and prescription drugs, and other environmental chemicals. The study consisted of 103 individuals who voluntarily enrolled in a detoxification program, and a control group of 19 individuals who did not participate in the program or receive any dietary instructions, exercise, or vitamin supplementation.

The participants started a detoxification program, which included: 20 to 30 minutes of aerobic exercise followed by 2½ to five hours daily of sauna at 140–180° F, nutritional supplements, increasing amounts of niacin to tolerance, water, salt and potassium replacements, two to eight tablespoons daily of polyunsaturated oil, supplemental calcium and magnesium, a regular schedule, sufficient rest and sleep. This program was followed for a three week period, with daily documentation of vitals and symptoms. In addition, physical examination, blood tests, and psychological testing were administered before and after participation in the detoxification regimen.

The test subjects had very few problems with the program, and were able to withstand the rigors of the exercise and long hours in the sauna. Although there were no measurable changes in weight during the program, it was noted that there were dramatic changes in blood pressure, and an 11 percent reduction in cholesterol levels, with triglyceride levels moving towards the mean from both low and high levels. The participants showed improvement in two-thirds of the physical complaints. There were statistically noticeable differences in the psychological testing before and after the program. The participants reported feeling better; they felt alert and able to think more clearly, they experienced an enhanced sense of smell and taste, and had more energy.

Previous studies had already shown that physical exercise hastens the metabolism of lipid tissue. The researchers felt this study showed that perspiration and sebum excretion allowed the xenobiotics released from the lipid tissue to exit the body, rather than being stored back in the lipid or muscle tissue. Since previous researchers have shown a correlation between stored xenobiotics and cancer, it would seem encouraging that there might now be a way to begin unburdening the body of these toxins. The study details discussion of the importance of vitamin and mineral replacements, adequate fluid, and the role of niacin in the program. The program was recommended as safe under the care of a physician, with careful and gradual increases in the physical exercise and sauna time.

It is notable that the references listed for this study contain 67 sources, many of which were previous studies of toxicity and sweat excretion of xenobiotics in various animals and humans from a variety of sources and countries. Finally, the researchers do not recommend this program for anyone with coronary artery disease or other serious physical disability unless under the immediate supervision of a physician who designs an exact program for the particular patient and provides immediate supervision.[20]

In 1983 Dan Christian Roehm studied a Vietnam veteran who had been exposed to Agent Orange and was showing the symptoms of exposure to DDE and PCB. Lipid analysis was performed for both of these chemicals before the veteran started a program of sauna detoxification. The detox regimen involved 39 consecutive days of the following: 15 minutes of aerobic exercise followed by 3¾ hours dry sauna, increased vitamin and mineral supplementation, calcium, magnesium, niacin, oils, and fluids. The symptoms related to DDE exposure resolved following the regimen. Adipose analysis showed an immediate reduction in both chemicals. Over the next 250 days following the sauna program, adipose stores of chemicals continued to decrease. Lipid analysis 250 days after the completion of the program showed a 97 percent reduction in DDE. The initial 27 percent reduction in PCB rose again following the initial decrease, most likely because of a recontamination of the same chemical.[21] This study suggests that sauna detoxification may heal the body's own ability to detoxify, and continue the detoxification process long after completion of the sauna program.

In 1984 Robert Amidon, a Los Angeles attorney, wrote an article for the *Journal of California Law Enforcement* bringing to light the stories of law enforcement officers who had been exposed to environmental contaminants on the job and were experiencing serious and disabling health consequences. His illustrations contained the following examples: a utility pole containing PCB downed in an electrical storm, the apprehension of a drug offender and contact with the substances, a fire or traffic accident involving hazardous wastes or chemicals. In his article, Amidon outlines the financial effect that disabled officers have on the State's economy, as well as the valuable loss of experienced personnel brought on by workplace exposures. He presented the Hubbard method of detoxification to officers and their families as a way they could be helped.[22]

A study published in 1984 brought together private and government researchers. David Schnare, Max Ben and Megan Shields chose seven healthy men who had participated in earlier studies on PBB contamination. These men participated in the Hubbard Purification Program for an average of 20 days. Adipose samples were obtained by removing lipid tissue through needle aspiration. Samples were taken three times: before and after the program and four months following the completion of the program. Of the 16 chemicals they analyzed, 13 were reduced, and seven of the 13 were significant. The reduction in chemicals averaged 21.3 percent, ranging from 3.5 to 47.2 percent. There did not appear to be any analytical error, nor could any of this reduction be attributed to loss of weight or fat during the program. As if these statistics were not impressive enough, the adipose tissue samples taken four months following the completion of the Hubbard program showed that all of the 16 chemicals were reduced, ranging between 10.1 and 65.9 percent, and averaging a reduction of 42.4 percent. This was an average additional reduction of 21.1 percent.[23]

In 1987 David Root, M.D., and Gerald Lionelli published a case report in the *Journal of Toxicology* about a woman, 23 years of age, who was experiencing medical complaints. She worked as a maintenance person, hosing the accumulated grime from a generator that was powered by oil. The medical personnel at work advised her to purchase and use safety equipment. She was treated by her family physician and sent back to work after two weeks. When she finally saw Dr. Root, she was experiencing low-grade fever, swollen lymph nodes, and acne. After treatment for mononucleosis and rest for two months, she returned to him with continuing lymph node enlargement, exhaustion, lethargy, and increased need for sleep. Three months later with the same complaints, her testing for specific infectious diseases being negative, she was diagnosed with low-level toxic poisoning, and participation in the Hubbard detoxification program was prescribed. Her program lasted 31 days. On the fourth day she began to excrete a black substance through her skin. This excretion continued throughout the sauna part of the program. Upon completion, her acne had cleared, the majority of her lymph nodes had returned to normal size, and her symptoms had abated. She was able to return to work, but was cautioned against further exposure to the oil and grime to which she had been exposed.[24]

In 1987, 14 firemen responded to a transformer explosion and fire. During the exhausting battle and clean-up, their protective equipment was either voluntarily removed or rendered ineffective. They had massive skin and inhalation contamination. Two to three months later all 14 men began to experience fatigue, weakness, joint pain and memory loss, among other symptoms. As time continued, some of the men experienced insomnia, difficulty with balance, and irritability.

These men were studied by Kaye Kilburn, M.D., Raphael Warsaw, and Megan Shields, M.D. The report was published in 1989. All 14 men participated in a detoxification program. The program they undertook consisted of exercise for 30–60 minutes followed by sauna. They completed this program twice a day, for two to three weeks. It is important to note that this study does not mention the length of time the firemen spent in the sauna, or the ratio of exercise to sauna, a factor previously deemed important in other studies.

The firemen were given an initial battery of neurophysiological and neuropsychological tests six months after the fire, and were given follow-up testing six weeks after participation in the two to three week detox program. The program resulted in improved cognitive function and memory. However, balance and choice reaction time scores became abnormal. Other tests remained unchanged. No correlation was found between the levels of PCB in their fat or serum, and their impairment. Most notably, the perception of the participant's own distress did not change or improve, even though the scores on several of their tests showed an improvement. The researchers concluded that it was not certain whether the detox regimen was successful. The improvement on the tests may have been due to learning from previous testing experience.

Questions were raised as to the possibility that the participating and control groups had experienced additional toxic exposures over the span of their careers, thus rendering this one exposure less significant.[25] Kaye Kilburn, M.D., writing an editorial in the same journal, questions whether perhaps the exposure of the firemen was "superimposed" upon years of previous exposures, and wonders what the results of the test would have been had the control subjects been without similar occupational exposures.[26]

In 1989 a controlled study of a group of persons exposed to PCB contamination was published. The scenario revolved around the small town of Semic, Yugoslavia. In 1961 Semic was a small town with 500 residents. Striving towards financial independence, a factory was located in the town which provided jobs for about 1,300 workers. Over the next ten years, the small town grew to 2,000 and eventually to over 5,000 residents.

The factory produced electric capacitors and used PCBs in the production process. In addition, the following chemicals known to cause medical problems were used: trichloroethylene, polychlorinated naphthalenes, and epoxides. The safety gear at the factory was ineffective. The employees, under strict demands for high performance, rarely used what little safety gear was available. The employees came into direct physical contact with the chemicals, and breathed the chemicals which were burned at the plant. Employees brought the chemicals home on their clothing to their families and often took their families to the factory for special dining privileges. In addition, PCB by-products were used in the homes and farms, and factory waste was dumped into the water supply and surrounding lands.

By 1984, following concern about PCB contamination of the new water system, and the discovery of malformed and sick fish, plants and produce, it became apparent that the contamination had spread to an area covering 50 square kilometers. This posed a direct threat to over 3,000 inhabitants and workers. Water samples at this time registered 600 times the United States limit imposed by the EPA for PCB in drinking water. As time progressed, the bitter public outcry of enraged citizens polarized government officials. Medical workers found that PCB serum levels of residents were ten times higher than expected for unexposed people. In addition, liver abnormalities, and other biochemical difficulties were found, as well as elevated enzyme levels, and other uncomfortable symptoms. The people were not improving despite various medical interventions. As the public demand for health care increased, and the budget of the socialistic medical system became strained, the government refused to recognize the town as a disaster area.

The story became more dramatic when one particular woman presented symptoms so serious as to require hospitalization. A local gastroenterologist recommended that she participate in the Hubbard detoxification program. A combination of government, factory and private American funds paid for her travel and treatment. Following the program, her symptoms abated and she had remarkable improvement. Upon her return to her homeland, her story spread to other ill workers. The public demand for treatment rose, and government officials tried to silence the woman and her children through harassment. The factory workers continued their demands for treatment. Finally it was agreed to appropriate funds for treatment of some of the other workers. Because of financial considerations, only 11 of the proposed 40 factory workers participated in the Hubbard detoxification program. Workers who were not treated provided a control group for the researchers. The chosen participants who were experiencing severe symptoms and physical difficulties, reduced their lipid stores of PCB and other chemicals after participation in the program. This benefited their immune system and helped alleviate their troublesome symptoms.[27]

Studies continue to be published about the positive results of sauna for many health problems. A recent database search on MEDLINE revealed 13 references on sauna and therapy from 1993 to 1996. Most of these studies concerned various applications of sauna for treating various heart conditions. Specifically they were

- a) temperature sensitivity managed by sauna (contrast temperature) treatment,
- b) hemodynamic improvement in congestive heart failure by sauna thermal vasodilation,
- c) sauna treatment for hypertensive patients,
- d) use of sauna for arterial hypertension,
- e) sauna and radon in treatment of arteriosclerosis obliterans,
- f) circulatory changes by use of sauna following heart transplantation,
- g) use of sauna in coronary heart disease, by-pass and aneurysm surgery.

One study was completed on the use of sauna on the clinical and psychological aspects of rheumatoid arthritis.

It is clear that disease is caused by occupational and environmental chemicals. Traditionally it has been difficult to diagnose and treat these illnesses. Even when people have been severely sick, traditional diagnostic tests and medical approaches have often not been helpful. This sometimes has led to a disbelief in the amount of physical suffering relayed by the patient, and a total disbelief and discounting of the patient's physical symptoms. High and low level chemical exposures have been shown to have documentable effects on the human system.[28] The studies reviewed above offer some hope for those suffering from toxic chemical exposures.

3. Understanding Detoxification

The Organs of Detoxification

The entire detoxification procedure is aimed at speeding up the elimination process through the major eliminating organs: the liver, bowel, kidneys, skin and lungs.

The Liver

The *liver* is a primary organ for processing vitamins and minerals and removing toxins. Chemicals mobilized through exercise and sauna enter the bloodstream where they pass through the liver. In order to help the liver do its job of cleansing and eliminating these toxins from the bloodstream, it is important to provide enough clean water so that the blood is continually being "flushed." Overburdening the liver with alcohol and contaminants only makes it work harder, thus decreasing its efficiency for eliminating other toxic materials. A chemically free water source is vitally important in this process of flushing out the toxins.

The Bowel

The *bowel*, a major organ of the digestive system, works in conjunction with the liver. Daily elimination is essential. If stool is not passed regularly, the toxins cannot be eliminated. If the toxins are not eliminated, then they are reabsorbed, re-enter the blood, are once again processed by the liver, and may be absorbed back into the tissues. The liver and the bowel can best work together by:

- A proper diet, high in fiber and nutrients, and low in contaminants, chemicals, additives and salt
- Lots of fresh uncontaminated water
- Regular elimination

The Kidneys

The *kidneys* are a major organ of the urinary tract. The main function of the kidneys is to cleanse the blood of waste products. These waste products are then passed on in the urine, and excreted from the body. At least two quarts of water are needed, daily, to enable the kidneys to do their job in flushing wastes and contaminants through the system, so that chemicals are not re-deposited back into our body tissues.

The Skin

The *skin* is another primary organ of chemical absorption and excretion. It has been found that the skin excretes an amount of toxin equal to the amount excreted in the urine.[29]

During exercise and sauna therapy the increased blood circulation and vasodilation causes increased sweating. In sweating, the hypothalamus activates millions of sweat glands located in the second and third layers of skin. Sweat is produced from the bottom coiled portion of the gland, and released through the glands' ducts. Once on the skin, evaporation provides a cooling effect.

As much as a gallon of sweat can be lost when exercising on a hot, humid day. The American Dietetic Association encourages athletes engaging in endurance events to drink:

- Three cups of water two hours before the event
- Two cups of water 10 to 15 minutes before the event
- One-half to one cup of water every 10 to 15 minutes during the event
- As much water after the event as needed, to regain whatever weight was lost through sweating.[30]

The skin, in order to do its job properly, needs regular care. It needs to be cleaned regularly with nontoxic soaps, protected from dryness with

safe oils and creams, kept from irritants by using a minimum of cosmetics, and kept dry and protected from the damaging effects of the
sun.

The Lungs

The *lungs* are the major organs of the respiratory system. After air
enters the body through the nose and the mouth, it flows through the
sinuses, which secrete mucous and are lined with cilia. Cilia are tiny
hair-like extensions from a cell surface. They perform a rhythmical,
wave-like action which carries particles and gases away from the lungs.
The cilia, and other cells that line the respiratory tract, protect the lungs
by absorbing 50 percent or more of the toxins we inhale. The remaining 50 percent that reaches the lungs may be stored on the lung lining
and cause further irritation, or may re-enter the bloodstream, be directed
to the liver, or be exhaled.

Breathing through the nose helps to protect the lungs, since the
nasal passages act as a filter to pollutants. The nasal passages can be
protected by breathing fresh clean air, uncontaminated by irritants or
toxins.

The body is an intricate mechanism designed to protect itself from
invading chemicals and foreign substances. The organs of detoxification
can do their job only with the proper environment. Proper food, nutrition, plenty of fresh water, clean air, daily rest, and regular elimination
are only the basics.

External and Internal Chemicals

Patients reacting to chemical exposures, react to two basic sources
of chemicals—external and internal chemicals.[31]

External chemicals are classified as those chemicals encountered outside of the body. These include the chemicals encountered in air, food,
water, living and working environments.

Internal chemicals are those chemicals we previously encountered
in the environment, and are now stored within the body's tissues. The
chemicals stored in the tissues of chemically ill people, are carried

around with them every day. These stored chemicals are the primary cause of the body's inability to handle additional external exposures.

To reduce external chemicals, each person must examine their living habits. The primary aim is to drastically reduce the toxins encountered in daily life.

The sauna detoxification program is aimed primarily at helping the body to excrete internal chemicals, the accumulated body-burden chemicals, those chemicals stored in the lipid tissues of the body.

A successful detoxification program must attempt to decrease both external and internal chemicals, not only by offering an intense exercise and sauna regimen, but also by controlling and modifying the total environment.

It would be pointless to enter into an exhaustive and expensive regimen of sauna therapy, only to inhabit an environment laden with smoke, mold or chemicals, and to eat food filled with additives, preservatives, and pesticides. The detoxification process works best with a combination of sauna therapy and strict environmental controls.

4. Getting Ready

Detoxification of Chemicals in the External Environment

The main purpose of the detoxification program is to help the body eliminate stored chemicals. Think carefully about every aspect of your life before beginning detoxification therapy. It is counterproductive to remove chemicals through the sauna process, and live in a chemical-laden environment, because chemicals can easily be reabsorbed back into the system. For detoxification programs to be successful, it is critical that the total environment be taken into consideration.

Grace Ziem, M.D. notes that patients with MCS often gradually improve if chemical exposures are reduced. She advises that it is important to control exposures at work, but especially in the home where most patients spend 10–20 hours a day.[32]

Depending on the severity of your illness and your own particular lifestyle, your environmental clean-up can be major or minor. By removing objects that "off-gas" (release in a gaseous form) chemicals into your environment, you may find that some of your symptoms clear on their own.

In any event, do not ignore this part of detoxification. Do not move on to the sauna and exercise program without taking care of these necessary steps. It may be helpful to begin with one area or room at a time. This will allow you to absorb the change, and to reduce your stress level. Anything that is overly stressful will not be helpful to you. Do what feels comfortable, what is affordable. Do only what feels right to you, only what *you* can handle.

The checklists that follow will help you think about the toxins in your living environment.

Pesticides

Look for pesticides in the following areas:

Spray cans
Fly spray
Ant and roach bait
Insect repellents
Pet flea and tick sprays, powders, collars
Moth crystals
Some shelf papers
Air fresheners (many contain para-dichlorobenzene)
Wool (contains mothproofing, which is often dieldrin)
Many commercial potting soils and mulches (contain pesticides and fungicides)

Neighboring lawn care practices
Agricultural acreage
Business or public areas that use ground treatments or ornamental controls
Restaurants and food stores
Commercial establishments
Schools
Cedar (although used as an alternative, is still found to be intolerable by many MCS people)

Petroleum Products

Petroleum is used in more products than you imagine. These are just a few:

Crude oil, motor oil
Rock oil
Paraffin oil and paraffin wax
Floor wax
Butane, ethane, propane
Naphtha
Gasoline, kerosene, diesel fuel
Asphalt
Ethylene, propylene
Alcohol
Ethylene glycols
Benzene
Phenol
Toluene, xylene

Pesticides
Paint thinner
Utility gas
Ink, ball-point and felt-tipped pens
Deodorizers
Cold creams
Mineral oil
Wax depilatories
Many cosmetics, lipsticks, rouge, eyeshadows, lipgloss
Petroleum jelly
Fertilizer
Furniture polish
Paints

Plastics—including shower curtains, lampshades, nonstick coatings on pots, left-over containers and food wraps

Synthetic fabrics—polyester, acrilon, rayon, nylon

Coal-Derived Chemicals

Coal tar is used in:

Adhesives
Creosotes
Insecticides
Phenols

Dyes
Hair dyes
Cosmetics

Combustion Products

Cigarette smoke
Candles
Wood fires and wood stoves

Petroleum or coal fuels for cooking, heating and clothes drying
Gas stoves

Formaldehyde

It has been estimated that 4 to 8 percent of the general population has been sensitized to formaldehyde. This list contains only a few common products which contain formaldehyde:

Disinfectants
Leather tanners
Defoamers
Preservatives
Rubber products
Dyes
Carpets
Adhesives
Mouthwashes
Nail polish
Wrinkle-proof and crease-resistant fabrics
Water-repellents and water-resistant finishes

Fabric softeners
Flame retardants
Pressed wood products
Plywood
Paneling
Particle and fiber board
Plastics
Paper products
Paper towels
Insulation materials
Combustion products (such as fuel exhaust and tobacco smoke)

A Practical Approach

The lists of chemicals in our home environment can be over-whelming. Many of us envision our homes as being "safe harbors" from chemicals. Because our homes do not contain noxious smokestacks, vehicle emissions, or heavy industrial contaminants, we imagine them to be safe.

Lately, however, indoor air has been the target of many studies. As early as 1962, Theron Randolph suggested that it might be more impor-tant to look at indoor air (as opposed to outdoor air) as a source of ill-ness in susceptible people. Twenty years later, his remarks were confirmed by others.[33]

With this in mind, we need to take seriously our responsibility for creating safe indoor air within our own homes and workspaces. When we spend eight to fourteen hours a day in our homes and a compara-ble amount of time in job facilities, it is logical that reducing air pol-lution in these areas is crucial.

The chemicals listed in the previous section, admittedly, are over-whelming at first glance. It can be confusing to tackle the job of clean-ing up an indoor environment by eliminating one chemical at a time. It might be far easier to break down the task by detoxifying one area at a time. It is often suggested to begin by detoxifying the bedroom, the room in which you spend a large amount of time within each 24 hour period. If you clean up just your bedroom, you have given yourself one safe room.

Once the bedroom is safe, it is easier to tackle other areas such as personal products, the kitchen, other living spaces and household areas, and environments outside of the home.

Bedroom

Keep the bedroom as simple as possible. Ideally, the bedroom should be bare except for a nontoxic bed, nontoxic bedding, a hard-wood, glass or metal nightstand, and a wood or metal radio, or alarm clock.

Street clothing and shoes should not be stored where you sleep. If it is possible, store your clothing and shoes in a separate room. If this is not possible because of space considerations, remove as much toxic material as you can.

You may want to invest in a carbon air filter, preferably one made specifically for the chemically sensitive. Whatever your situation and your choices, it is important to have this room, where you spend at least 30 percent of your time, be as safe as possible. Consider the following:

- Remove any mattress containing foam, synthetics, flame retardants, or insect repellents. Replace with untreated cloth mattress or futon.
- Remove synthetic or plastic mattress covers and pads. Replace with cotton mattress pad, barrier cloth mattress covers and untreated cotton sheets and blankets.
- Remove synthetic and wool blankets, even if they say "nonallergenic." Replace with 100 percent untreated cotton.
- Remove foam rubber, polyester and polyurethane pillows, cushions and other accessories. Replace with 100 percent cotton pillows, untreated organic wool or feathers, if tolerated.
- Remove any furniture containing plywood or pressboard. Replace with hardwood, glass, or metal.
- Remove synthetic drapes and curtains. Use metal blinds, or 100 percent untreated cotton curtains. Beware of fabric finishes that are perma-pressed, crease-resistant, or easy-care, since they contain formaldehyde.
- Remove rugs that contain rubber or jute backing, are synthetic, or mothproofed. Remove all rug pads. Consider using only washable cotton scatter rugs.
- Remove books, bookcases, and shelving units which collect dust. Try to keep the room uncluttered and bare.
- Remove all cosmetics, perfume bottles, deodorants, scented products, plastic accessories, plastic lamps, lampshades, picture frames, and all cardboard.
- Remove plastic garment and storage bags.
- Check the inside of all drawers and closets for scented sachet.
- Use no furniture polish or wax in this room.
- Make sure that only 100% cotton clothing is stored in closets and drawers. Remove leather, wool, synthetic, or vinyl clothing, shoes, or handbags, and all furs.

Personal Products

This is the hardest area for many people to tackle. Often self-image and esteem are linked with personal and beauty routines and products. Unfortunately, many of the personal products people use to help make themselves feel better often actually make them sicker. It is easy to deny that the face cream cherished and used for many years may be the reason behind the edema or acne that cannot be controlled. It is hard to imagine that a product used for many years could now be suspect, or even possibly damaging to one's health. The area of personal products and clothing are the most difficult arenas to change.

The skin is an organ of the body.[34] Contrary to what many people think, the skin is not an impenetrable surface. Rather, it easily absorbs chemicals that surround it and which are applied to it. What we apply to our skin is absorbed right into our bodies. A safe rule-of-thumb is, If it can be eaten, then it may be safe to put on your skin. If it is organic, and nontoxic enough to be ingested through the mouth, then it may be safe to attempt to ingest it through the skin.

The simplest way to evaluate the safety of our personal-use items is to simply *stop* using *all* cosmetics and personal products for a brief time. Perhaps your dry, itching, flaky skin, or the rash on your face or underarms will stop once you stop using your moisturizer, soap, astringent, or deodorant. You can get cleaner than you think with just warm water and a wash cloth.

While you allow your skin to enjoy this "vacation," you can do several things:

- Carefully check the ingredients of all previous products. They should not contain fragrances, dyes, preservatives, formaldehyde or petroleum products.
- Locate a book on cosmetic ingredients, and begin to learn about the common chemicals found in personal products. Educate yourself. Find safe and nontoxic alternatives. Explore new products. Locate some of the many home recipes for moisturizers, conditioners, and cleansers. Collect information and catalogues.
- Remind yourself how absolutely attractive you are without your chemical additives! If you are one of those people who feel charming only because of your make-up, after-shave, mousse

or hairspray, then this may be difficult. Expand your own personal definition of true "beauty." Learn to love yourself as you are.

- Talk with others who have located and who use safe, nontoxic, fragrance-free products. Ask them for small samples, so you can test the products for yourself.
- Make a list of what alternatives you may like to try.
- Indulge yourself. You are definitely worth it.
- Introduce new products *one at a time*. Give your body a few days to adjust to each new product and to monitor your reaction. Do not go too fast. Pay attention to any local or systemic reaction that may develop.

In addition, the following tips may be helpful as you redo your wardrobe and collection of personal products:

- Most fragrances, colognes and perfumes are toxic and contain long lists of hazardous chemicals. Some individuals cannot tolerate "essential oils" purchased from health food stores, or "aromatherapy."
- Avoid aerosol sprays.
- Volatile compounds that evaporate easily, such as nail polish removers and hairspray, are very damaging. Pay particular attention to mousse, hair gel, hair permanents, dyes, colorings, and setting lotions. They are particularly noxious.
- Plastic combs, brushes, and barrettes, and clips with plastic coatings and ends can be irritating to the scalp.
- Some dress shields contain plastic liners which may be irritating.
- Many feminine hygiene products contain scents and preservatives.
- Menstrual pads often contain deodorants, formaldehyde, bleach and other chemicals. Try a chemical-free brand, disposable cotton pads, or washable cotton menstrual pads. Some women use a folded bandanna or diaper. Tampons often contain chlorine and deodorants. Some have been found to contain dioxin.
- Toilet tissue can contain dyes, fragrances and chemicals. Locate an unbleached, fragrance-free alternative.
- Plastic eyeglasses, lenses or contact lenses may cause itching, dark circles, and dryness. Metal or graphite frames, polycarbonate lenses, and nylon or silicone nose pads may be an alternative.

- Toothpaste often contains dyes, fragrances, glycerin, formaldehyde, and flavorings. Try plain baking soda, or baking soda mixed with salt as an alternative.
- Some people are sensitive to different types of plastic pens and inks. Try pencils, metal pens, unscented ink. Also available are "anti-gravity" pens, which write upside-down, and can be useful when sick in bed, or writing while lying down.
- Many people have difficulty with a variety of paper products and scented stationery. Recycled, nonbleached papers and paper bleached with hydrogen peroxide are now available.
- You may want to invest in a carbon water filter for your shower or tub to eliminate chlorine and other chemicals. Make certain to replace the filter units regularly.
- Vinyl and plastic shower curtains are not recommended. Replace with 100 percent cotton duck curtain.
- Prescription drugs contain petrochemicals, dyes, coatings, preservatives, and tableting agents. Some specialized pharmacies compound special formulas without these additives, under a physician's direction. Often these come in the form of "pure powders," which can be put in gel capsules and kept in the refrigerator. There are also alternative herbal remedies and nutritional supplements available for specific problems. Get professional advice.
- Products containing menthol, camphor, or eucalyptus are often irritating.
- Chemically sensitive people often cannot tolerate synthetics. This includes polyester and cotton-polyester blends. Even wool is often not tolerated, because most wool is moth-proofed with pesticides. Cotton, linen, natural rayon and silk seem to be the most easily tolerated. Some people have difficulty with the dyes, bleaches, finishes, or pesticide residuals on commercial cotton fabric. Try unbleached muslin, "green cotton," or organic cotton.
- Locate 100 percent cotton clothing, that does not have drip-dry, crease-resistant, stain-resistant, or wrinkle-proof formaldehyde finishes.
- Some people tolerate articles that have been dry-cleaned and are well aired; others may not.
- Consider not using chlorine bleach, antistatic dryer sheets, and fabric softeners. Sizing and spray starch are also particularly irritating.

• Be careful about new detergents marketed as fragrance-free. Often these "fragrance-free" products are the same perfumed product, with the addition of an "odor masking agent," "olfactory masking agent," or nasal anesthesia.

Food and Kitchen

The food we put into our systems provides the nourishment that feeds, sustains, and repairs the cells of our bodies. If we put processed, sweetened, pesticide-contaminated, artificial, preserved food into our system, we are polluting our bodies.

Since the turn of the century, farming as a way of life has been steadily declining. Today, about 98 percent of our food is grown by huge corporations that fill our food with pharmaceuticals, pesticides, preservatives, and petrochemicals.[35]

Food is grown in overworked soil, fed with artificial fertilizers, injected with artificial hormones and growth stimulators. It is then processed, bleached, colored, preserved, watered-down, packaged, irradiated, fumigated, thawed, and marketed.

For the chemically sensitive person, food is a vital issue. Taking care in the selection, purchasing, storing and preparing of our foods, is vital to our healing. Debra Lynn Dadd, in her *Non-Toxic, Natural and Earthwise*, suggests these things:

• Eat fresh foods that are not processed.
• Buy foods that are organically grown.
• Eat foods that are locally grown and common to your geographic area.
• Cut back on meat consumption. Eat only meats that are raised without harmful chemicals. Eat more vegetables.
• Start your own garden.[36]

Certified organically grown food is more expensive and is sometimes difficult to find. What you are paying for is food grown without synthetic fertilizers, pesticides, herbicides, fungicides, antibiotics, other drugs, and hormones. Make certain that the food is packaged without chemical additives.

Try to buy only food marketed as "Certified Organically Grown." Do not be misled by food labels that use the term "organic" or "unsprayed" and may not meet the requirements you need to properly protect your health. This is an individual decision that depends upon the level of your sensitivities to pesticides and other additives. In addition, some of the following tips may be beneficial, and worth considering:

- Consider some avoidance trials to determine food sensitivities.
- Find out what foods make you sick. There are many books to consult on pinpointing food allergies. It has been suggested that foods which are craved often point to a hidden food allergy.
- Consider a rotation diet.
- Consider vegetarianism or macrobiotics.
- Avoid alcohol.
- Purchase food not packaged in heat-sealed containers, or tin cans which leach phenolated can liner and lead into food. Some processors of organic food use a preferable enamel lining in their cans.
- Repackage all food in cellophane, cloth or glass for storage.
- Cook with an electric stove, hot plate, electric skillet, electric wok, or crock pot.
- Do not use pans and cookware with nonstick coatings.
- Avoid plastic utensils, storage containers, or microwaveable cookware.
- Use iron, stainless steel, glass, or Corning Ware for cooking. Aluminum is not recommended.
- Keep all foods in covered, closed containers. Do not risk a pest infestation.
- Keep the kitchen clean and well ventilated.
- Run a ventilator fan or open a window when cooking. If possible, shut the door to the kitchen, so cooking odors do not permeate the house.
- The kitchen is often one of the most polluted rooms in the house. With a wide array of products, appliances, and heavy use, this area needs to be kept as clean and well-ventilated as possible.
- Check under the sink and remove any toxic cleansers and cleaners which may be off-gassing.

- Do not use chlorinated tap water for drinking or cooking.
- Bottled spring water is only as pure as the spring from which it came.
- Distilled water stored in plastic containers contains plasticizers which leach into the water.
- Consider a home water distilling unit, or a reverse-osmosis water filter, for your drinking and cooking water.

Other Household Suggestions

- Store vehicle maintenance supplies (oil, antifreeze, etc.) in a shed or garage away from the house.
- Remove any yard and garden products, pesticides, weed control or fertilizers.
- Ask for assistance in cleaning the basement, garage, or other areas of the house, and removing all toxic substances from your living space. Do not forget turpentine, paint, bleach, ammonia, and other popular household disinfectants.
- Be aware that building products can be toxic. Plywood, pressboard, and some insulation products contain formaldehyde. Pressure-treated lumber also contains harmful chemicals.
- Remove the disinfectant pad located in the mouthpieces of many telephones. Cover plastic phone receivers with cotton covers, or locate metal telephones. Speaker phones are widely used.
- Provide ventilation, for proper fresh air exchange. This can be done in many ways, from expensive filtered ventilation systems, to simply opening the windows on a periodic basis.
- Operate room air filters throughout the house. A variety of filtration media are available. Samples for testing can be obtained from many filter manufacturers.
- Avoid commercial floral arrangements and potted plants. Commercial potting soil often contains pesticides.
- Many electrical motors, audiovisual equipment and computers outgas plastics and other chemicals. Try to locate these appliances in areas of your home that you use minimally. Provide ample ventilation, exhaust or filtration in the areas where these appliances are located, and especially when they are in use. Another alternative is to locate part of each appliance in your living

space and another part in a closet, adjoining room, basement or attic. For example, you may choose to locate the computer monitor and keyboard in your work area and the central processing unit and printer elsewhere. You may choose to locate the speakers to your stereo in your living room and the components in the closet. On the other hand, some people have grouped all of their appliances together, enclosed them and provided ventilation to the outdoors.

- Keep coats, boots, shoes, and miscellaneous street items out of your living space, if possible. Leather, plastic, and vinyl out-gas hazardous chemicals, and outer garments often bring in contaminants from the out-of-doors.

- Upholstered furniture often contains dust-mites, molds, and bacteria. In addition, synthetic cushions and fabrics, stain-repellents and fabric finishes all out-gas fumes. Replace with hardwood or metal furnishings, if possible, and natural cotton upholstering.

- Remove as much printed material, books, magazines, newspapers, files, etc., from your living space as possible. Store elsewhere. Use glass or metal enclosed bookcases for necessary books.

- Remove wall-to-wall carpets, rug pads, paneling, draperies, synthetic cushions, curtains and window shades.

- It may be impossible to rehabilitate some buildings because of the presence of persistent pesticides. Some particular pesticides are known to have a half-life of 25 years or more in soil. No one knows exactly what the half-life of certain pesticides may be indoors, without the presence of sunlight and other weather conditions to break down the chemical.

Community Hazards

- Avoid gas stations. Ask a friend to fill your tank, or pay extra for "full service." In some states, a handicapped license plate entitles the driver to have free assistance by service station operators. Check out the laws for your locality.

- Other areas that may be hazardous to your health include: dry cleaning establishments, landfills, sources of industrial emissions, commercial and public places that use lawn care, pesticides, agricultural or grounds treatments, shopping malls, etc.

- Investigate your state department of agriculture to see if you have a registry for pesticide sensitive individuals. If not, perhaps you can become involved in having one established. These registries mandate that pesticide sensitive individuals be notified by commercial pesticide/herbicide applicators prior to lawn treatments.

- Request neighbors and adjacent properties to notify you prior to pesticide applications and other projects that involve the use of pesticides, petroleum products, and other noxious chemicals.

- Inquire about municipal spraying programs in your area for mosquitoes, gypsy moths, and other pests common to your locale.

- Avoid rush hour, heavy traffic areas, freeways and tunnels; use less-congested routes.

- Try not to drive behind busses and trucks.

- Consider purchasing a 12-volt carbon air filter for your car, which plugs into the cigarette lighter. Some severely ill have also found success using carbon respirator masks, portable oxygen, or a combination while traveling.

- Avoid parking garages.

- Obtain a handicap license tag or sticker for adjacent parking to avoid traffic fumes and parking garages.

- Get to know the merchants in your area, and work with them to adapt to your needs. Use the phone to shop. Perhaps, if you call ahead, merchants can bring the items out to your car, or mail or deliver purchases to you. Some have found a car phone useful in soliciting the help of merchants for curbside service. Others have difficulty with the high electromagnetic frequency of cellular phones.

- Get a supply of catalogs for other purchases. Plan ahead. Keep the catalogs stored in a place apart from your immediate air-space.

- Commercial and home swimming pools are highly toxic to many individuals. A few pools are now being sanitized with hydrogen peroxide or benzalkonium chloride, rather than chlorine, although some people are still reactive to the algaecide used with these products. Many fresh and salt water bathing areas are contaminated with *E. coli*, and the run-off of pesticides from adjacent agricultural lands. In addition, many municipalities treat their lakes, ponds, and reservoirs with algaecides and fungicides.

Work Hazards

- The Americans with Disabilities Act of 1990 requires employers to provide reasonable accommodations to persons with disabilities.
- Request prior notification in writing for any pesticide application, building repairs or maintenance.
- Request the above to be done on Fridays, or before holidays, so off-gassing can occur while you are not in the building.
- Inform the building management, in writing, about Integrated Pest Management, and other low cost, less-toxic methods of building maintenance.
- Request ventilation for your work areas. Different localities have various standards for minimum air exchanges per hour. Investigate.
- Consider purchasing, or have your employer purchase, a charcoal filtering device for your office or work area. Make certain it is one specifically designed for the chemically sensitive, that it does not contain particleboard, plastics, chemical components, or off-gas contaminants.

These lists are only intended to be a sampling of ideas to help you protect yourself and clean up your environment. For additional information, consult the reference material at the end of this book.

5. Deciding: The Options

The Programs

L. Ron Hubbard began using sauna detoxification in the early 1970s with persons addicted to LSD and other street drugs. The success of his program led to its use with alcoholics and those suffering from the side effects of prescription drugs and medications. Twenty years later, there are many detoxification programs available. Many physicians, specialists, physical therapists, toxicologists, and spa administrators have developed their own specific formats for the detoxification process.

Ashford and Miller list the seven basic components of most detoxification programs:

1. Twenty to thirty minutes of aerobic exercise
2. Two to five hours of low temperature sauna (140 to 180°F)
3. Nutritional supplements, with increasing amounts, including niacin
4. Replacement of lost water, salt and potassium
5. Two to eight tablespoons per day of polyunsaturated oil
6. Additional calcium and magnesium
7. Daily exercise and sauna, completed in a routine with regular meals and rest.[37]

Each of these factors has equal weight in importance for the success of the program. Positive results cannot be expected if any facet is left out, minimized, or ignored. It is the *total program* that has made sauna detoxification a viable health tool for many people with multiple chemical sensitivities.

Detoxification programs vary in their approach. Below are two examples

The Hubbard Method

L. Ron Hubbard is known, among other things, for his "Hubbard Method," or "Purification Program." In his book, *Clear Body, Clear Mind: The Effective Purification Program,* Hubbard describes his methodology in a detailed and definitive format. In the introduction to the book, Megan Shields, M.D., describes the etiology of his program and her experience with the program through her extensive research. The book contains a thorough discussion of the role of exercise, particular information on sauna, charts and lists of vitamin, mineral, magnesium, calcium, oil and niacin supplementation, and other pertinent information.

Bridge Publications offers a companion guide, *Purification Rundown Delivery Manual,* based on Hubbard's work.[38] This manual is a daily log for the person participating in the Purification Program, and provides checklists, medical report forms, daily forms and other information helpful to the participant. Gene Denk, M.D., writing an evaluation of the Purification Program at the beginning of the manual, details his experience with the Hubbard program. He, in conjunction with several other colleagues, published a study that was the result of detailed testing of the Hubbard Purification Program on 103 volunteers.[39] Hubbard's program entails:

1. Exercise—running to increase circulation and release of waste
2. Regular sessions in the sauna—140 to 180°F
3. A ratio of approximately 20–30 minutes running and 4–4½ hours of sauna
4. Regular daily schedule—including necessary rest and sleep
5. The program continues daily for two to three weeks, depending on individual tolerance
6. A partner is necessary, for safety, at all times
7. Sufficient (copious) fluids[40]

8. Proper nutrition—including plenty of fresh vegetables

9. Vitamin and mineral supplementation—exact regimen of vitamins, minerals, and trace minerals, including salt and potassium supplements, with a blend of fresh cold-pressed polyunsaturated oils, and lecithin. Hubbard's book provides detailed charts with specific quantities and measured increases of niacin, calcium, magnesium and other supplements, in an easy-to-follow format.[41]

10. Regular blood pressure and other tests completed at regular intervals.

The Hubbard Method is offered at "Health Med," formerly in San Francisco, and currently in Sacramento, California. The program is strenuous and should only be started following a thorough physical examination and written approval from a medical doctor.

The Environmental Health Center

The Environmental Health Center, in Dallas, Texas, was founded in 1974 by William J. Rea, M.D., and the American Environmental Health Foundation, Inc. The Center offers a wide variety of diagnostic and treatment services. Their concentrated physical therapy program offers exercise, dry sauna, massage, vitamin, mineral, and oil supplementation. Patients requesting information receive detailed instruction on the use of specific personal products, proper clothing and suggestions on locating safe housing prior to arriving in Dallas.

Before participating in their programs, an initial history, physical, and assorted blood assays are given, as well as tests to detect the presence of pesticides or volatile chemicals in the blood.[42]

Each day's program begins with taking vital signs, and the administering of niacin to individual tolerance. Exercise, sauna, shower, and massage constitute one session. A normal day consists of three sessions for a total of four to five hours. Before leaving the unit, each patient is given vitamins, minerals, oils, and other supplements as determined by individual need.

The program is administered by a physician, nurse, and physical therapist. Blood levels are monitored each week, in addition to other lab work prescribed on an individual basis. The program continues six days a week, for four to six weeks, and may be longer depending upon individual need.[43]

*   *   *

Sauna detoxification centers are located all over the country, and around the world. Each of them have certain similarities and important differences. Do your own research. Ask questions. Locate people who have finished the programs and ask about their experiences. In addition, consider the following:

- Find a physician who cares, listens, and understands MCS and who responds to your questions.
- Seek out health professionals who successfully treat other MCS patients.
- Locate a support group. Sometimes this takes the form of telephone networking. Ask others to share their knowledge and experience with you.
- Read as much as you can on MCS, different methods of treating it, and articles written by people working in the field.

Personal Stories

The following are personal stories of individual experiences with detoxification centers and home saunas, as told to the author. All names and places have been changed. These stories serve to illustrate the successes as well as the frustrations and disappointments that can be encountered.

Case 1

Anne B. lived close to a major detoxification center. She was very chemically sensitive. She decided to attend the center at the recommendation of her doctor. She drove herself to and from the center each day, and arranged assistance for transportation on those days when she was not feeling well enough to drive. She spent five to six hours a day, seven days a week, at the center, for 55 days.

While undergoing the program, she stated that she was so tired and exhausted that she often had to rely on fast food for meals. This was the only difficulty she encountered during the program.

She met many wonderful people and gained new information. Blood tests before and after the program showed significant changes in Candida and antibodies. Her insurance paid 100 percent of her treatment. She improved dramatically, and maintains her health with a careful diet, regular sweat baths, exercise, and yoga.

Case 2

Calvin D. was very sick when he decided to fly to an out-of-state detox center. The air travel exacerbated his illness. When he arrived, he discovered that accommodations were not safe for his sensitivities, but was determined to continue with the program. His frustrations were increased as his illness made him unable to shop for his own food or take care of himself outside the treatment facility. He could not tolerate the preservatives and colorings in the required mineral drink. He became too sick to continue the program and returned home.

Case 3

Elizabeth F. had tried everything to get better. Sauna detoxification was her last-ditch effort. She prepared by switching to a macrobiotic diet, and removing toxins from her home. She traveled to a detoxification center, where she completed the rigorous program in 60 days.

Upon her return home, she had a serious relapse, because she could not locate a safe sauna in which to continue her maintenance program. Her condition continued to deteriorate. She decided to have a sauna built in her home and began taking saunas daily, until her health improved. She returned to the detoxification center, and again completed the program. This time, when she returned home, she was able to continue the maintenance regimen in her own home sauna unit. She continues to improve.

Case 4

Gary H. had severe allergies and asthma, in addition to his MCS. His doctor often prescribed prednisone to quiet his symptoms. While on this medication, he was able to safely travel to an out-of-state detox center. Once there he weaned himself from the drug, and successfully completed the program. He is now able to go to the mall, restaurants, and take short vacations without serious reactions.

Case 5

Ivan J. was becoming increasingly sensitive to chemicals at home and at work. He felt he needed to do something before he became sicker. As the sole financial support for his family, he could not afford to be ill. He read about sauna detoxification and decided to try it.

He purchased a membership at a local health club. Regularly after work, he took time to exercise and sauna. Even though he encountered soaps, aftershave and deodorants in the locker room, he believed the benefits of the sauna far outweighed the effects of these exposures.

Several months later, the health club began renovations. Despite his worsening condition, he was determined to continue his program. After successive days of increased dizziness, nausea, and continued exacerbation of his illness, he collapsed during a workout. As he was being removed to the hospital, he questioned the health club staff about any chemicals used in the building. He was informed that a roach infestation had been discovered during the renovations. The entire building had been treated with pesticides.

Unfortunately, Ivan became disabled from this pesticide exposure, and subsequently lost his job.

Case 6

Kathy L. attended a detox center and reported feeling very "clean" when she left, but also very sick. Her condition had deteriorated even though other MCS people in attendance noticed benefits from the program. Five years later, her condition has improved, but she does not attribute her regained health to her detoxification experience.

Case 7

Margaret N. experienced an array of serious symptoms upon exposure to chemicals. She decided to attend a detoxification center. Early in the program her physical condition deteriorated. She was too ill to return home and was hospitalized. She was diagnosed with an underlying heart condition, and underwent cardiac surgery. After a lengthy recuperative period, she returned to the detox center, and began the detoxification process. Her condition improved and she successfully completed the program. Her insurance reimbursed 80 percent of her costs. Upon her return home, she continued the maintenance program at a local sauna and attributes her current state of health to "sweating out" the toxins at the center.

Case 8

Oliver P. did not want to travel out of state to a detox center; he preferred, instead, to spend his money on a sauna which he could use for the rest of his life.

He took a year to research and test the materials for the construction of his sauna. He contracted a carpenter to build it to his specifications.

The sauna was installed in his basement, along with exercise equipment he purchased for use in his home program. A ventilation system was installed that pulled fresh air in through a window filter, through a second filter in the sauna, and vented the stale air from the sauna to the outside. He removed toxins from his home and purchased air filters for use in each room.

His program includes 30 minutes of aerobic exercise, followed by a 40 minute sauna, five days a week. In addition, he takes niacin, oil, and other supplements as prescribed by his doctor. He maintains a strict organic diet. The laboratory comes to his home, periodically, to draw blood for laboratory analysis.

After a six month period of regular exercise and sauna his health has slowly and steadily improved. Oliver is convinced that he made the correct choice.

*   *   *

These personal accounts reflect a wide variety of experience. In general, people are willing to share their experiences with others in similar situations. Learning from the experience of others is one valuable tool in the research process. You might want to imagine yourself in any one of the above situations, and try to imagine how you could have foreseen the problems, or changed the situation to protect your own health. It is important to be very clear about your own health status and situation, and set realistic goals. If you make decisions to protect yourself, you will maximize your chances of success.

So, Now What?

Many doctors recommend sauna therapy to their patients. Armed with little more than this advice, the patient is often bewildered about where to turn next. Perhaps you are thinking about undertaking a sauna detoxification regimen. Either you have read about the benefits, you have had a friend share their "success" story with you, or it has been recommended to you by your doctor or other health professional.

Some questions you may be asking are: Where would I take a sauna? Should I attend a detox center? Should I purchase a sauna? These are important questions to ask. There are many different solutions to each question, and to each person's particular situation.

Very sensitive individuals experience extreme health repercussions with the introduction of *one new item* into their environment. As a chemically sensitive person, you know how long it took to locate a safe shampoo or detergent. The cost of many unused bottles of shampoo is minimal when compared to the expense of a sauna experience.

Perhaps you have changed to a macrobiotic, vegetarian, organic or rotation diet. You are aware that this took reading, planning, talking with others, trial and error, and a real commitment to make it work. Just like beginning a new dietary regimen, entering the realm of sauna detoxification requires a similar willingness to take responsibility for investigating all the aspects, and a determination to make it work.

With this in mind, it is easy to expect that entering into a sauna experience will require much thorough research and planning. Be careful in your research. Everyone's sensitivities are different. What is sold, marketed or even *guaranteed* as safe for chemically sensitive individuals *may not be safe for you.*

Many patients hope that saunas will cure them. They yearn to continue with their lives as they used to be, and will try any reasonable approach.

Some people *do* improve with sauna detoxification. Others may not. Most people find that saunas are a wonderful tool for *gradually* improving their health, over a period of time.

Just as people make different choices about integrating new diets into their lives, people make different choices about the *format* of their sauna experience. Some people go to a detox center for one program, others return a second time, and some attend at regular intervals. Some people purchase home saunas, and use them daily, or several times a day, for short or long periods of time. Then there are those who use a combination of attendance at detox centers for the in-depth program, and the use of home saunas for the follow-up maintenance program.

Go slow. Ask many questions. Do not expect to call a specific company, order a sauna, have it delivered, plug it in, take a sauna, and feel better that evening! Likewise, you cannot expect to make an appointment, travel to a new city, and begin the program without careful consideration and advanced planning.

The *best* chances of success are with those people who carefully plan and research their options, who continue their research all along the way, and are willing to "shift gears" if something isn't working as planned.

Gather the facts. Ask a lot of questions. If things go wrong, you have a lot to lose. If you take time to research and plan carefully, you may have much to gain!

A Closer Look at the Options

Examine the following questions and considerations as you explore the possibilities available to you with sauna detoxification therapy.

Local Health Clubs

The saunas at local spas, gyms, YMCA, or health clubs are readily available to anyone living near an urban area. With a basic membership, you can often use the exercise equipment, in addition to the dry saunas or steam baths.

If you choose this route, think through every possible chemical which you might encounter. Remember, a health club is not an establishment for the chemically sensitive, and not all saunas are safe for the chemically sensitive. It will depend on the particular club or facility, the willingness of the personnel to accommodate your needs and answer your questions, your own particular health status and what chemicals trigger your reactions as to whether or not using a health club sauna is a safe choice for you. Consider the following list of questions:

- Does the health club use pesticides regularly? Do they subcontract with an outside agency for pest control?
- Do they have carpeting?
- What building materials have been used in the construction of the sauna? Some chemically sensitive persons have difficulty with traditional cedar or redwood saunas, others do not.
- What insulation is used in the sauna? If you are very sensitive to formaldehyde, this could be a very important question.
- Are bathers required to shower before entering the sauna?
- Will the fragrances lingering on the bathers also linger in the sauna?
- Is the sauna ventilated?
- Are bathers allowed to use oil, creams, lotions, or hair conditioners while using the sauna?
- What products are used to clean and disinfect the sauna?
- What about the locker rooms and bathrooms? Will soaps, personal products, disinfectants and deodorizers be a problem for you?
- Is there a ventilation system for the entire building? Get the details.
- Is there any construction or renovation occurring within the building? Are there plans for this in the near future?
- Is someone nearby to help in an emergency or if you become ill while on the premises?

If you are considering sauna therapy because of chemical sensitivities, then consider the potential harm to you by regularly encountering all of the chemicals within the health club. You may be able to communicate with the administrative staff, and be forewarned of the presence of any chemical contaminants. It may be safer to use the sauna at a time when the bather load is low.

Weigh all the pros and cons. Talk with your physician. You do not need to risk another chemical injury. On the other hand, why pass up an inexpensive and readily available sauna, if it is safe and convenient?

The Detox Center

Sauna detoxification centers are springing up across the country. Some are geared to a population of substance abusers, recovering alcoholics, and health impaired clients, while others cater specifically to the chemically sensitive population.

If you are considering traveling to a center for treatment, think carefully through every facet of your travel, your treatment, and your accommodations. Do not be embarrassed to ask even the most rudimentary questions, especially about food, water, and air! Your health is at stake, and only you are responsible for it. Any reputable detox center that deals regularly with chemically sensitive people will understand and welcome your questions. In fact, they will probably have special staff assigned to handle all your questions, and the details of your visit. Some guidelines to assist you before calling a detoxification center are:

- How can I travel to and from the center? Can I use oxygen en route?
- Will someone be able to travel with me, and physically assist me during the program?
- Who will help me if I become ill?
- Where will I stay? Are pesticides used?
- What if I cannot tolerate the housing provided? What other accommodations are available?
- Are there stores nearby which offer organic food and fresh organic produce?
- If I am not able to shop for my own food, will someone be able to assist me?
- What about laundry facilities during my stay?
- What is the water like? Is it filtered? How?
- What happens if I become too ill to cook, shop, and care for myself?

- What is the center like? Is the building built with materials which are less toxic?
- Are the sauna and physical therapy areas clear of structural and other chemical contaminants that would threaten my success?
- What type of sauna is available for my use? Are there sealants, glues, or other toxins in the sauna? Does the insulation contain formaldehyde? Is the sauna cleaned with harsh disinfectants and deodorizers?
- What comprises the exercise part of the program? Is suitable equipment available for my use? Is there fresh air and adequate ventilation? Wall-to-wall carpeting?
- What is the daily and weekly schedule for my program?
- What are the hours of the program? Will I be traveling during heavily polluted rush-hour times? How will I get to my temporary residence if I am too ill to drive or navigate by myself?
- What rules apply to personnel and other participants with whom I may have contact? Will they use personal products that might hamper my success?
- What types of laboratory analyses will be required? Where will I be receiving my laboratory tests?
- What types of medication, supplements, vitamins, and oil will I be expected to consume? Are they free of agents that are sensitizing to me? Do they contain preservatives, additives, or colorings? What are the possible side effects of these supplements? Is the staff willing to modify this aspect of the program to meet my specific needs?
- Who is in charge? What is the training and experience of the personnel? Will I have access to emergency medical care?
- Is there an M.D. on the staff?
- What is the ratio of clientele to professional personnel?
- What is available to me in terms of 24 hour health care? What options are available to me if I become ill after leaving the center, or at night? Who can I call in an emergency?
- Are there any previous patients with whom I can speak?
- Are there patient support groups?
- Is psychotherapy available for any emotional problems that may arise during the course of my sauna therapy?

- What are the costs and fees of the program? Are there any additional costs? Will insurance, or Medicare cover my treatment?
- What can I expect after the program is completed? Is care available for me following the program, if needed?
- What type of maintenance program is recommended once I return home?

Home Sauna Units

It may be that you are not able to safely travel to a center, or tolerate accommodations outside your home. You may not feel that you can care for yourself in a strange city without a support person, or your support person may not be able to travel with you. Perhaps your insurance will not cover the detoxification program. It may be easier to obtain the necessary assistance, safe food and water, and medical attention that you need while remaining in your own home.

For all of these reasons, and others, you may decide that it does not feel right for you to travel to a detox center. Perhaps, for you, the investment in a home sauna unit may be a safer and more economically feasible approach. With the investment in a home sauna unit, you can attempt the detoxification process at a slower, less rigorous rate, and for a longer period of time. In fact, with the ownership of a sauna, you will have the increased advantage of having this type of detoxification available to you on a permanent basis. For many reasons, building a home sauna may be a preferred approach.

In addition, many detox centers require a maintenance program that includes three to five saunas per week, after leaving the center. Some people combine attendance at a detox center, with the purchase of a home sauna unit, for ongoing treatment. The installation of a home sauna unit can be a valuable tool for home detoxification alone, or in conjunction with other sauna programs. The home sauna unit can be a long-lasting part of a daily health regimen, geared at not only obtaining but maintaining an optimal level of health.

6. Home Sauna Units

What to Consider: The First Steps

If you are considering purchasing a sauna for home use, it is necessary to consider every facet of your total environment, your medical and health needs and goals, as well as your financial situation. Examine the following:

- Do you own your own home, or do you rent?
- Do you want a sauna that is permanently installed in your home, a small portable sauna you can easily transport to a new apartment, or a larger prefab unit which can be disassembled and reinstalled in a new dwelling, should you choose to move. (These differences will be discussed in greater detail later in this chapter.)
- Where do you plan to locate the sauna? Outside? In the basement, spare room, living room, garage, or porch?
- What type of electrical hook-up is available for the sauna heating unit? If you live in an apartment, or rented home, you most likely need a heater that can simply plug into a standard 110-volt outlet. This will limit the size of the heater and sauna. If you own your own home, you have the option of installing a separate electrical circuit, which will power a larger heating unit. A larger heater can heat more square feet of sauna to desired temperatures.
- How many bathers will be using the sauna? How many at one time? Do you envision yourself sitting up, or reclining? Do you have difficulty sitting in one position for long periods of time? Some small units provide only enough limited space for one bather

69

in a sitting position. Others, require the bather to recline. Larger units allow the bather the option to sit or recline.

- What are your budgetary constraints? Do you want to invest in a smaller unit to see how sauna therapy works for you? Others with sauna experience and committed to sauna therapy, may feel inclined to invest more money in the purchase of a larger sauna unit.

- How much time do you plan to spend in the sauna? What does your doctor advise? Will you be doing long detox programs with three to five hours of daily saunas, or only shorter maintenance saunas? The number of hours you plan to spend in the unit will help to determine what type of structure you need to ensure your comfort. Some people feel faint with exposures to higher temperatures and need to lie down. The vasodilation that happens with heat exposure sometimes causes the blood pressure to fall. Some persons with low blood pressure find it necessary to lie down while in the sauna, and sit up only at intervals to change positions or drink fluids. Those who find heat difficult to tolerate, often find with regular sauna therapy that not only do they become healthier and thus better able to withstand the heat but their bodies acclimate and adjust to the temperatures.

- Check with your local building authorities to find out any county or municipal regulations governing the building of saunas. Building codes, or "codes" as they are commonly called, set standards for the design and construction of buildings, additions, and sometimes even parts of buildings such as saunas. These codes cover the materials, electrical wiring and other facets of construction. In some locations you may need a building permit to build a sauna within or adjacent to your home. If you are planning to build your sauna outdoors, check to see if any zoning regulations may apply.

There are a variety of sauna models on the market made out of various materials, with an array of options. The basic components will be outlined in the following sections.

It is not the purpose of this book to make any recommendation or to endorse any specific products. The purpose of this book is to set forth the options and the various positive and negative considerations to assist you in making your own choices. As with the purchase of any other piece of medical apparatus, you are best advised to discuss your ideas and needs with your physician(s). Talk with others, test all products, and proceed slowly.

Basic Components of the Sauna

A sauna is another room in your house. If you were building another room, or an addition to your pre-existing home, you would be concerned about the foundation, flooring material, framing, wiring, insulation, and other details about the room. These same considerations are important when considering building or purchasing a home sauna unit. For a chemically sensitive person, these considerations are even more vital, and require a great deal of forethought, testing and planning.

For the purposes of this section, we will consider the two basic components of a sauna: the enclosure and the heat source.

The Box, or Enclosure

The enclosure, box, or sauna itself, can be made of many different materials: ceramic tile, wood, glass, metal, or fabric.

Ceramic Tile Saunas

Ceramic tile has the advantage of being inert, and extremely safe for those with severe MCS. It has the distinct disadvantage of being very heavy, and expensive to install. A ceramic tile sauna is not considered a "portable" or "pre-fab" unit after installation.

The saunas in use at the Environmental Health Center in Dallas, Texas, are made of ceramic tile. The tile covers the floor, walls and ceiling of the saunas.[44] Portland cement is often recommended, with sand and water used to set the tiles. Adhesives and mastics are *not* recommended.

Wood Saunas

Wood is often recommended as a second choice for sauna construction, if tile is not desired. Wood is not only easier to work with, it has the advantage of being lighter and providing the possibility of assembly, disassembly, and reassembly.

Some people can tolerate the resins in wood, others cannot. If the wood sauna is to be located in a living space where you spend a great deal of time, this may be a serious consideration. Some people have noticed an increased sensitivity to wood and wood products, following the installation of a wood sauna that was located in their main living area. Others find that they can tolerate the resins if the wood is located away from their primary living space. Locating the sauna in a basement, garage, or a room separate from the house, with adequate ventilation, may help protect from over-exposure to wood resins.

Any unsealed wood has an odor. Air or kiln-dried lumber has less odor than fresh cut wood. Over time, odor diminishes, as the resin in the wood dries. During a sauna, the outward convection of heat causes odors to flow outward. (*See Illustration 1.*)

As the sauna cools, the dropping temperature reverses the heat convection, thus pulling the heat and wood odors back into the compartment. For this reason, a wood sauna will have more wood odor inside the sauna when the unit is cool, and more wood odor outside the sauna while the unit is operating. (*See Illustration 2.*)

For these reasons it is important to consider:

• Your general tolerance of wood and the specific wood you are considering for your sauna.
• The location of the sauna. If the sauna is located in your immediate living space, the odor may be more noticeable than if it is located in a separate room.

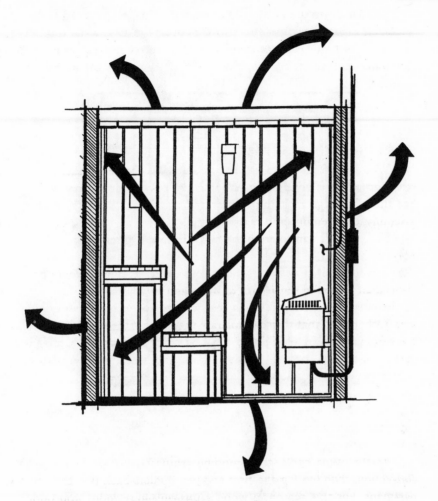

1. Outward convection of heat energy

- The presence of other persons while the sauna is in use. Will the odors of the warm wood bother you, or someone else, while the sauna is heating up and while it is in use?
- A ventilation system is a possible remedy. This will be discussed later in this chapter.

The major factor to consider when selecting a particular wood for use in constructing a sauna is the amount of resin in the wood.

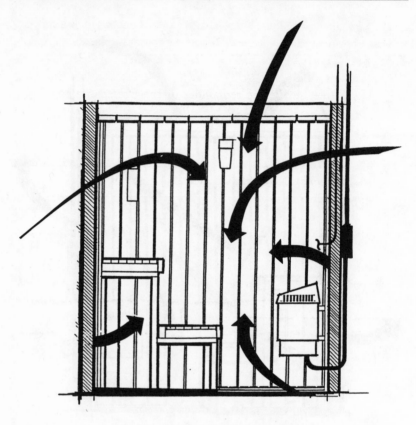

2. Inward convection of heat energy

More resin means a greater degree of aroma from the wood. What determines the amount of resin is the moisture content of the wood. Any laboratory can test for this. A wood with a 10 percent moisture content is a good choice, 8 percent being better, and 12 percent being less desirable.

Redwood and cedar are often used for construction of saunas but are *not* recommended for those with MCS because they contain the highest amount of resin. Western hemlock and basswood are sometimes suggested, although there are those who complain of lingering odors from these two types of wood.

Poplar is generally believed to have the least amount of resin, and it is well-tolerated by many (although not all) MCS sufferers. For this reason, it is often recommended. Poplar is a deciduous fast-growing tree of the genus *Populus*. There are many varieties of poplar, including black poplar, cottonwood, and aspen. Different geographic locations refer to different trees as being "poplar." For instance, when referring to poplar, the Canadians mean aspen. People from the Great Lakes region mean the "popple tree," while the remainder of the United States assumes yellow poplar. Commercial poplar is yellow poplar. The sapwood (outer sides of the inner tree) of the yellow poplar is known as white poplar, and gives up its resin, or sap content easily. Aspen and white poplar are particularly low in moisture content and preferred by many chemically sensitive individuals for use in wood saunas.[45]

Kiln-drying the wood before use decreases the moisture content, and aids in off-gassing the resin, saps and tree odors. If possible, this is well worth the extra cost. Different kilns use different fuels (gas or wood) to dry their lumber. Ask questions.

If you decide to use wood, it is important to test it first. Many companies will gladly send you a sample piece of wood, about 4" × 4" × 1". This is *not enough* wood to accurately test your reaction to this particular type of wood. Request or purchase several pieces of the lumber, and freshly cut the lumber into smaller blocks, to release the fresh resins. Then,

- Spend time with it, keep it near you, see how you do.
- Sleep with it next to you, or keep it on the bedside table.
- Put it in the oven, in a glass casserole, or on a layer of aluminum foil, and bake it at 140° to 180°F (normal sauna temperatures) for about 30 minutes. Be aware of odors coming from the oven, or from the wood after it is removed from the oven.

Glass and Metal Saunas

Glass and metal saunas are less expensive than ceramic tile saunas, and provide an excellent alternative for those persons sensitive to wood. Furthermore, they provide the option of being able to be disassembled and re-assembled.

A small glass greenhouse with metal studs can be purchased commercially, and modified for use as a sauna. Clean all glass and aluminum with dilute white vinegar to remove manufacturing residues. The glass panels in the roof and next to the heater can be replaced with tempered glass to insure safety. The heater can be purchased separately, and be freestanding, or mounted on wood attached to a wall. Dennyfoil™ vapor barrier (a brand of double-sided heavy gauge aluminum foil used specifically by the environmentally ill) can be applied to the glass of the greenhouse, to provide a reflective insulation, and to insure some privacy.[46] See the Appendix at the end of this book for more information on specific products mentioned throughout this text.

Some companies are currently marketing special order saunas made from a combination of glass and metal. Although metal conducts heat, it is durable and could be feasible when used for certain panels of the sauna with the addition of wooden guardrails for protection.

Fabric Saunas

Fabric saunas are an answer to the need for inexpensive, small, extremely lightweight and portable sauna units. One commercially marketed unit consists of a frame made of heat tempered aluminum L-bars, covered with undyed, unbleached, untreated cotton, and a heater. The bather enters the unit through a zippered door. The cotton covering is removable and washable, and may be dried on the aluminum frame.[47]

A Homemade Sauna

In an effort to save money, some MCS patients have designed and constructed their own units. For example, one person designed a homemade sauna using an old white oak playpen for the exterior frame. The bottom and side slats were removed. A bench was fashioned of oak and placed inside the structure. A cotton drape of untreated cotton canvas, covered the participant, whose head stuck out, and formed a "tent" over the playpen. (*See Illustration 3.*)

Untreated cotton canvas, or duck, is available from many catalogues specializing in products for the chemically sensitive. The person who designed this homemade sauna obtained the cotton canvas from a hardware store where it was packaged and marketed as a painter's untreated cotton drop cloth. With repeated washings it worked quite nicely. An opening was cut in the fabric for the head, and drapery weights were sewn into the bottom hem to keep the "tent" from lofting or billowing

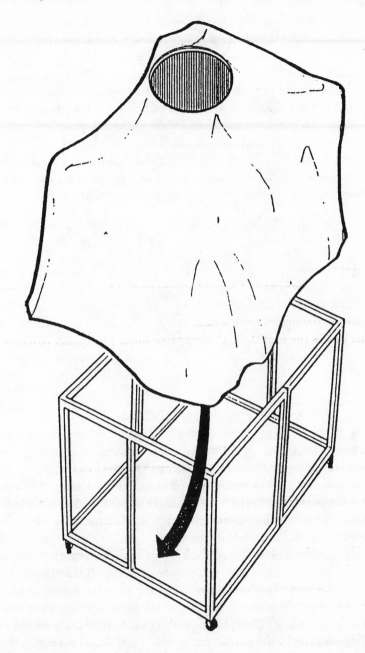

3. *Homemade sauna unit*

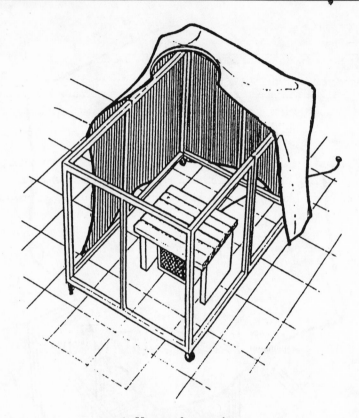

4. Homemade sauna in use

during use. To prevent neck chafing, a cotton terry towel was wrapped around the neck prior to donning the canvas tent sauna.

A porcelain radiant heater was placed *under* the bench. This position of the heater was found to be the most favorable because the bench provided protection from the heating unit, and because the heat was not generated directly on the body, causing problems with the drying of skin and mucous membranes. An inexpensive space heater was used. Because most space heaters are set to normal room temperatures, the thermostat was removed to allow the heater to heat to higher sauna temperatures. An oven thermometer was placed on the bench. The thermometer was monitored until the desired setting was reached, whereupon the participant entered the unit by lifting the "tent" and climbing in. This homemade sauna is collapsible and easy to store.[48] (*See Illustration 4.*)

Flooring

The foundation and floor of your sauna are largely determined by the location of the sauna. If you are planning to locate your sauna outdoors, you will need to construct a floor with masonry and framing construction (either wood or metal), which will resist frost and moisture. If you are building or locating your sauna indoors, the flooring considerations will probably be less difficult. Even though the floor is the coolest spot in a heated sauna, it is important that the material chosen for the flooring be safe and nontoxic when heated above normal room temperatures. Durability, moisture resistance and sanitation are other important considerations. The flooring most often recommended is ceramic tile, cement, or wood. Wooden duckboards, can be fashioned from a safe wood (poplar) and are made of wood framing with strips of

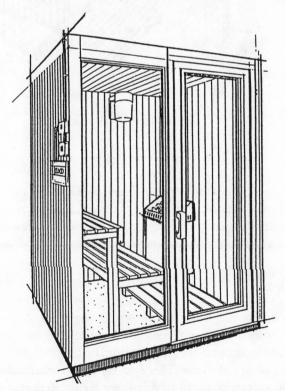

5. Fully assembled sauna unit (see prefab vs. fully assembled sauna units)

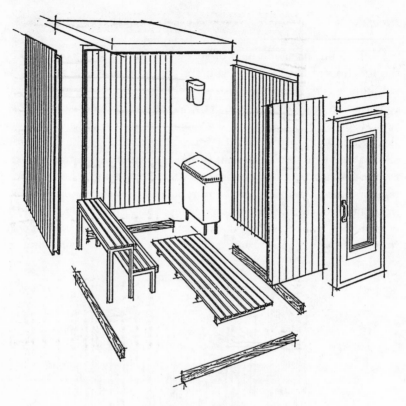

6. Prefab sauna: Exploded view

wood attached, similar to decking. These duckboards can be placed over a sealed concrete floor, and are easy to place and remove for cleaning. Be certain that any concrete flooring is sealed with a safe masonry sealer. Carpet or vinyl flooring is not recommended.

Hardware

The hardware used to put the sauna together must be considered for toxicity, durability, and resistance to moisture. Many metal hardware items come coated with a petroleum oil finish, to protect the product from rust or corrosion. This coating can be scrubbed off with any safe, nontoxic cleanser, and air dried thoroughly. Repeated washing and airings may be necessary.

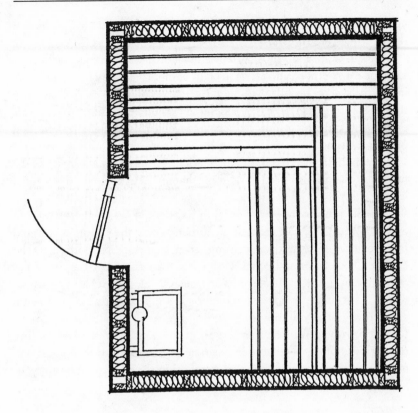

7. Prefab sauna: View from top

Galvanized steel nails are zinc plated, and sometimes difficult to use. Regular steel hardware may rust, or may be treated with rust resistant finishes. Brass screws have a tendency to strip easily. Brass-plated hardware may not be as durable as other choices, and may erode and allow rust. Although expensive, stainless steel may be considered the best choice.

Safe lighting fixtures are also available, constructed of porcelain, stainless steel, aluminum, or glass.

Prefab vs. Fully Assembled Sauna Units

Fully assembled sauna units arrive in one large box, already assembled and ready to use. These saunas are smaller units, weighing approximately 150 to 250 pounds. They are similar in design to a telephone booth, and often arrive collapsed, folded-up, or in sections that fit easily together. (*See Illustration 5.*)

Prefab saunas are most often larger units, weighing approximately 1,000 pounds or more, and arrive in eight or more separate cartons, depending on the size of the unit. Although the makers of these "kits" often claim that these units can be easily assembled in one evening, this depends on the skill and strength of the persons involved, as well as the definition of "one evening." You might like to have someone who is adept with tools, and physically able to lift the sections of the sauna assist you in the process. You will also need basic tools: hammer, drill, screwdriver, and a level.

Prefab saunas are constructed in large heavy wall panels which fit onto a floor frame, and are held by joiners. After the ceiling is lowered into position and the door is hung, trim is added, in addition to the benches, the heater and other accessories. (*See Illustrations 6 and 7.*)

It is important to do some basic research before purchasing a sauna, whether it comes already assembled or is a prefab unit. The following section will assist you in understanding the materials, design and other factors involved in the construction of a sauna. Understanding the various options available in basic sauna construction will assist you in asking the right questions and purchasing the correct sauna for you.

Heaters

Historically, saunas were heated using wood or coal stoves. Heat is a form of energy. All substances, whether animal, vegetable, or mineral, radiate heat. This heat flows by three methods:

- Conduction—the direct flow of heat through solids or gasses by actual physical contact.
- Convection—the transfer of heat in a gas or liquid caused by the flow of the gas or liquid itself.
- Radiation—the transmission through space of energy, by means of infrared or heat rays.[49]

All three types of heat are used in saunas. For the chemically sensitive, two basic types of heaters are considered safe, convective and radiant. (*See Illustration 8.*)

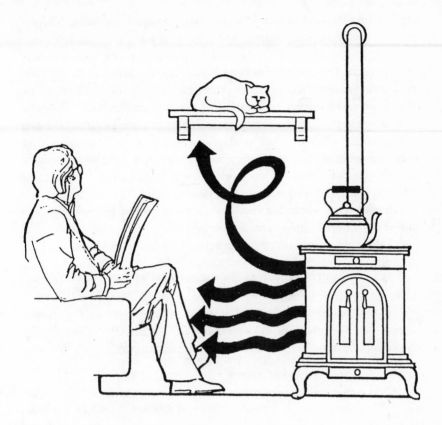

8. Heat energy

Convective Heaters—Convection heating systems work on the principal of warming the air, which in turn warms the objects in the room. In a traditional convective heater, an electric coil housed in a metal box heats up to a high degree. In a convective sauna heater, the electric coils heat the air that flows through the unit while heating the sauna rocks. The sauna rocks then provide a conductive heat source of their own. Cool air is pulled up through the unit and warmed by the coils and the rocks as it continues to rise towards the ceiling. As the air cools, it sinks to the floor and is then reheated and cycled throughout the room. This type of heater creates sauna temperatures from 140° to 180°F.

Radiant Heaters—Radiant heaters transfer infrared rays which directly warm objects much like the sun's own heat. These units are usually smaller, and run on less electricity. Normal operating temperatures for saunas using radiant heaters are between 110° and 135°F.

The choice of which type of heater to use is a very personal choice, and is crucial to your happiness with your sauna. Many people are convinced that radiant heat provides a more even distribution of heat within the room, and a deeper penetration of heat within the body. They feel this causes better blood circulation, and more profuse sweating at lower temperatures. On the other hand, many people are very unhappy with their radiant heaters, and feel they cannot work up a good sweat, because the temperatures just are not high enough. The choice is a personal one. Some companies, realizing this, offer a choice. What is best is what is safe and what works for you. Try various types of heaters. See how you react. There is no correct answer.

Other considerations when purchasing a sauna stove are

- Is the heater constructed of a material that will not out-gas, preferably one made of stainless steel, baked enamel or aluminum?
- Do you want a floor-mounted or wall-mounted unit? Floor-mounted units are usually more powerful, and carry a greater weight of sauna rock, which causes better performance. Wall-mounted units, however, may be more suitable for units where space is a consideration.
- How long will it take the stove to preheat the sauna to desired temperatures? Thirty to 45 minutes is considered a reasonable time.
- Does the heater meet Underwriters Laboratories (UL) standards? Does the manufacturer guarantee it? Can it be repaired locally?
- How long can you expect the stove/heater to function under the extremes of heat and humidity that it will operate?
- Will you need to install a separate circuit to power the unit? Will you need to bring 220-volt service to the sauna? The saunas powered by 110-volt service are designed for smaller one or two person units. For anything larger than this, powering a 110-volt heater can be ineffective and costly. For any electrical wiring that is required, be certain to hire the services of a competent and licensed electrician who knows the electrical and building codes for your jurisdiction.

Electric conductive heaters usually feature coils that are arranged in a fashion so that the sauna rocks can come in direct contact with the heating elements. It is important that the rocks have direct contact with the heater coils, so that the rocks stay hotter for a longer period of time, assisting in maintaining the temperature of the sauna. The rocks should be packed in the heater coils in such a fashion as to allow the heat to circulate among them, with the larger rocks on the bottom, and smaller ones on top. The saunas that provide trays on top of the unit for holding the rocks do not allow the rocks to come into contact with the heater coils and are less efficient.

Sauna rocks are important in maintaining the temperature of the room. Once the rocks are thoroughly heated, they store heat and generate it back into the room. The rocks usually used in saunas contain large pieces of igneous granite. These rocks are often from Finland where they are formed by centuries of heat and pressure. They can withstand the heat without splitting and cracking. With regular use the rocks will need to be replaced after several years.

Many companies coat their heater coils with oil, as a rust-preventive. Some people have difficulty with this oil coating. Others have difficulty with the lava rocks. A good soaking in sodium hexametaphosphate, tri-sodium phosphate, or baking soda, as well as a thorough scrubbing and a few days baking in the sun, can often help eliminate either of these problems. In addition, the initial "curing" of the sauna (described later in this chapter) will assist in out-gassing any impurities in the rocks or heater coils.

It is important to select the right size heater for your sauna. There are a variety of radiant and convective sauna heaters available, measured by the kilowatts used to heat them. Saunas located outdoors in the winter will obviously require a more powerful heater than a smaller sauna located indoors year round. In general, it is safe to calculate one kilowatt for each 45 cubic feet of interior sauna space. To calculate this, multiply the length × width × depth of your sauna. Take this number (for example: 6' × 6' × 6' = 216 cubic feet) and divide by 45 (216 divided by 45 = 4.8). A 4.8 kilowatt stove would be adequate for a sauna this size, unless you were locating the sauna outdoors and wanted to use it during the cold months.

Electrical Wiring

Most sauna units that are fully assembled and designed for one or two persons use a 110-volt heater and plug directly into household

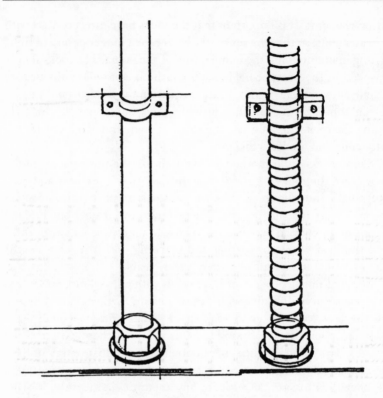

9. Electrical conduit

current. Larger and prefab units require wiring at the manufacturer, and some degree of electrical wiring upon assembly.

The wiring for the sauna must be able to withstand sauna temperatures over 180°, and withstand the constant change of temperature and moisture as well. Heat-resistant plastic coated Romex™ wire is usually run inside of the metal flexible conduit, or metal rigid conduit. Plastic conduit, even if it is heat resistant, is not recommended. The wiring should be located in the walls of the unit, behind the insulating material or reflective barrier. Another option is to have the wiring located on the exterior of the unit, inside rigid metal conduit. (*See Illustration 9.*)

The parts requiring wiring include the heater/stove, control box, thermostat, and light. Be sure to use all-metal heat resistant conduit, metal controls, and metal junction boxes. The switches should be located

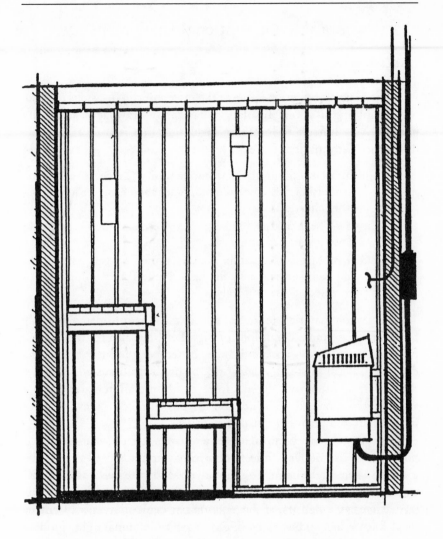

10. Exterior or intra-wall wiring of prefab sauna

on the exterior of the sauna. All metal parts should be cleaned prior to installation, for removal of manufacturing oils, dirt and dust. In addition, make certain that oil is not put on the wires as they are pulled through the conduit. A licensed electrician can wire the sauna "to code" for your particular jurisdiction. State laws vary considerably, as to wire sizes, conduit sizes, and electrical safety codes. (*See Illustration 10.*)

Considering Optional Equipment

Insulation

The issue of insulation is one of the most difficult decisions to make when building a sauna. Insulation has many drawbacks, primarily because it is difficult to locate an insulation that is truly safe. Basic difficulties with insulation are

- Chemicals—Most insulations contain formaldehyde and adhesives. In addition they contain mold, rodent and flame-proofing, and other chemicals.
- Fibers—The inhalation of fiberglass and ceramic fibers is known to cause respiratory problems.
- Other problems—Insulation materials often attract pests, molds and moisture, and are a fire hazard unless chemicals are added to remedy these problems.

Insulation materials for use in saunas must be considered not only for their safety under conditions of high heat, but also for their moisture resistance, since extreme changes in temperature may cause condensation. Because of these demands, the products discussed below are the ones most often considered. However, all insulation materials pose some degree of hazard, and while this can be controlled somewhat, careful thought and planning must be stressed.

Air Krete™ is a pumped-in cementitious foam insulation, and is nontoxic. A dye derived from natural clay sources is used to give the product a blue-green color. The pink dye used in the past has been discontinued, making this product very inert and nontoxic. Because this insulation has a density of 2.0 pounds per cubic foot, it may not be ideal for use in building lightweight or portable saunas. This product has, however, been used with overwhelming success in the construction of homes by many chemically sensitive people, and would be ideal for use in tile or permanent saunas.

Cerablanket™ insulation (Thermal Ceramics Inc.) is made of spun ceramic fibers, which are woven into a pad-type blanket. It is composed of alumina, silica, and small amounts of calcium oxide and magnesium oxide, and is very low-odor. Cerablanket™ insulation was designed for insulating furnaces and heating ductwork; it works very well for the high temperatures of saunas. Although woven ceramic fibers have not been approved by the government, the industry has placed voluntary restrictions on the use and application of this product. The problem lies with air-borne respirable ceramic fibers which may become lodged in the lungs and cause health problems. Rather than an MCS individual handling this product, it might be advisable to hire a worker who could use appropriate respiratory and safety gear. A number of MCS people have successfully been able to tolerate Cerablanket™ insulation by having it encapsulated inside bags of Dennyfoil™ vapor barrier. These bags are taped shut with Polyken™ 337 foil tape. The foil provides a barrier to the lofting of ceramic fibers, and makes this a possible choice. (*See Illustration 11.*)

Another way of using the foil to encapsulate the insulation, is to attach the foil inside the framing lumber. To do this, lay the exterior wall section, consisting of the framing lumber and exterior wall, on the floor. The framing lumber will create a cavity, which when completed will be the interior wall space. Into this cavity, place a sheet of Dennyfoil™ vapor barrier. Cover the entire cavity, and staple it to the framing lumber. Lay the insulation on top of the Dennyfoil™ vapor barrier, and cover it with another layer of Dennyfoil™ vapor barrier. Staple the second layer of Dennyfoil™ vapor barrier in place, and seal with Polyken™ 337 foil tape. Finally, attach the next section of framing lumber, and interior wall. This process of encapsulating the insulation secures all particles inside the Dennyfoil™ vapor barrier. The Dennyfoil™ vapor barrier is secured by being stapled, taped, and held firmly in place between the two pieces of framing lumber. (*See Illustration 12.*)

Dennyfoil™ vapor barrier is a double-sided aluminum foil on Kraft paper facing. It can be used as a foil vapor barrier insulation, by itself, or in conjunction with other insulating materials. When installed, it is necessary to provide an air space between the foil and the walls, to prevent moisture buildup, and also to reflect the heat back into the sauna interior. The Denny Corporation, or certain distributors (such as Foust Co.) can provide brochures showing the proper installation of a foil vapor barrier.

Polyken™ tape is an aluminum foil tape, and is often used in con junction with Dennyfoil™ vapor barrier, for various purposes. It can be obtained locally through building and hardware stores. Polyken™ offers many varieties of foil tapes. Make certain that you select Polyken™ #337, and not #339, or other similar tapes. The difference lies in the

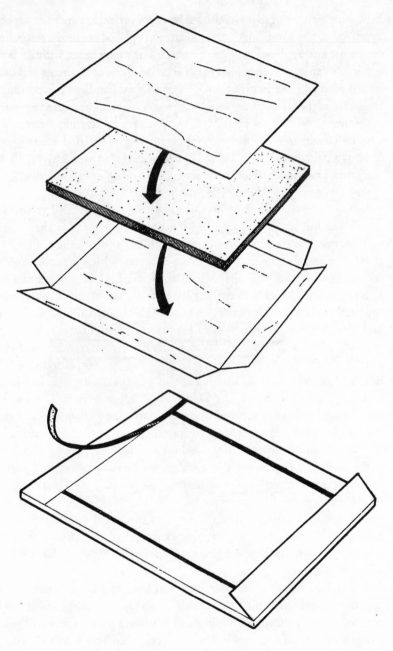

11. Foil bags of insulation

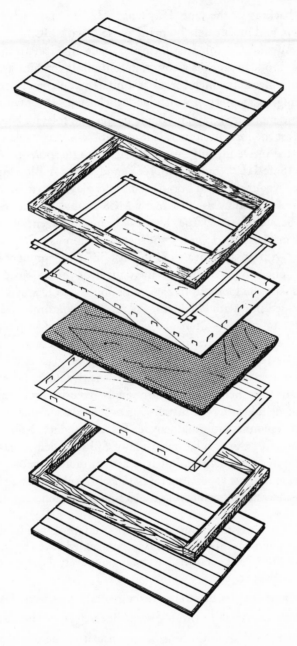

12. Foil encapsulation of insulation within frame of sauna

adhesive backing of the tape. Polyken™ #337 foil tape has been used most often, and most safely by many persons with MCS.

Greenwood Cotton Insulation™ made by Greenwood Cotton Insulation Products, Inc., is a cotton insulation. It contains a small percentage of polyester, which serves as a binder, and comes with a Kraft paper facing, in a variety of widths and thicknesses. It contains boron as a flame and moisture retardant. Some people can tolerate boron, others cannot. Test the insulation first. If it is a problem, the insulation can be encapsulated in Dennyfoil™ vapor barrier. (*See Illustrations 11 and 12.*)

InsulSafe III™ (by CertainTeed) and **Class A Blowing Insulation™** (by Knauf) are two brands of fibrous glass blown-in insulation. They have been safely used by many MCS people, and are considered nontoxic because they lack the chemicals or binding agents used in other fiberglass insulations. However, the lofting of fibrous particles has been connected with possible health problems. Since this product is chemically safe, one way to counteract the danger of the fibrous particles is to encapsulate the loose fill in bags of double-sided Dennyfoil™ vapor barrier, sealed shut with Polyken™ foil tape. (*See Illustrations 11 and 12.*) These bags, or "pillows," of insulation can be mounted within the walls, much in the same way that traditional batts of insulation are installed.

CertainTeed™ makes several brands of fiberglass batt insulation, which have been used by some chemically sensitive individuals who consider it safe for them. Other individuals have become sensitive to formaldehyde following the installation of fiberglass insulation containing minute amounts of formaldehyde. Test all products before use. The encapsulation of this insulation inside of foil may help to contain the off-gassing of formaldehyde, but it is always more difficult to contain the emission of toxic vapors than it is to keep fibers out of an air space.

Consider the following when selecting insulation:

- Call or write the companies mentioned (see Appendix for further information) or any others recommended to you by friends with MCS. New products are coming out every day. Investigate and ask questions.
- Request samples, literature, pricing, and Material Safety Data Sheets.
- When the samples arrive, test them. Be careful not to inhale any fibers.
- When working with these or any insulating materials, *obtain and use a heavy-duty industrial respirator that contains the proper*

cartridge for fibrous materials. Any manufacturer or salesperson can discuss this with you. *It is vital to your safety and health.* Because of the dangers inherent in many insulating materials, it is advisable to hire a worker to handle the insulation. Anyone using insulating materials should use proper respiratory and safety equipment.

• "R" value is a rating which describes the insulation's ability to stop the flow of heat through the material. The higher the number of the rating, the better the insulation is for colder temperatures and extreme fluctuations in temperature and humidity. An "R" value between 11 and 19 is considered average for exterior walls. Local laws and codes may vary. Foil vapor barriers do have an "R" value, and this rating can be increased by applying the foil to allow an air space.

• As a last resort, consider not using any insulation at all. The old-fashioned saunas, built outside and used in winter temperatures, often had no insulation, and were considered quite effective.

If you take the time to collect the data and test the products, it will become clear to you which insulation, if any, is preferable for you.

Ventilation

All saunas need some type of ventilation to provide fresh air. Without a steady and adequate supply of fresh air, the bathers in the sauna will not have the necessary oxygen and humidity to breathe easily. It is crucial that the hot stale air from inside the sauna have a way to escape. This hot dry air can become very irritating to the respiratory passages without the steady influx of fresh, moist air. Many saunas do not supply adequate ventilation. A properly designed ventilation system will not unnecessarily waste heat, nor will it cause uncomfortable drafts.

The ventilation system may be active or passive, with the air filtered or unfiltered.

Passive Ventilation—commercial saunas located in public establishments and those marketed for home use often use a form of *passive ventilation.* One major manufacturer of saunas, recommends that the air be exchanged six times an hour. Passive ventilation can be provided in several ways:

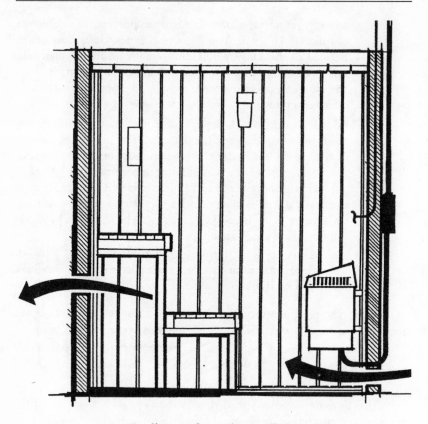

13. Air vents for passive ventilation

- Cut the door an inch or two shorter to allow fresh air to enter beneath the door.
- Open the door momentarily, when fresh air is desired.
- Cut an opening in the wall directly below the heater for incoming air. Cut an air outlet opposite the heater, about two feet higher than the incoming vent, but lower than the upper benches. The flow of heat will cause the air to circulate as cool air comes in, rises, and flows out the vent. (*See Illustration 13.*)
- Some people feel more comfortable with filtered incoming air. A simple way to do this would be to cut an opening near the floor, the dimensions of a standard size air filter, and merely insert the filter into this space. You can use either a HEPA, charcoal filter, or any filter of your choice. For example, if HEPA

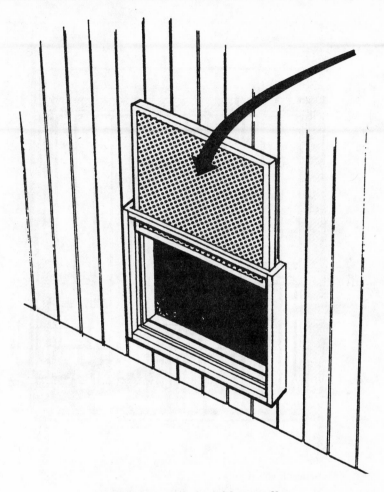

14. *Passive ventilation with HEPA filter*

filtration is desired, cut the opening approximately 8½" × 12",
the size of the HEPA filter that comes with Allermed's Airstar
5-C™ air filter, and use their HEPA filters as replacements. Any
other filter can be used, with appropriate adjustments made. (*See
Illustration 14.*)

Active Ventilation—An active ventilation system may be desired
to provide a more frequent exchange of air. Some ideas for achieving a
system of active ventilation include:

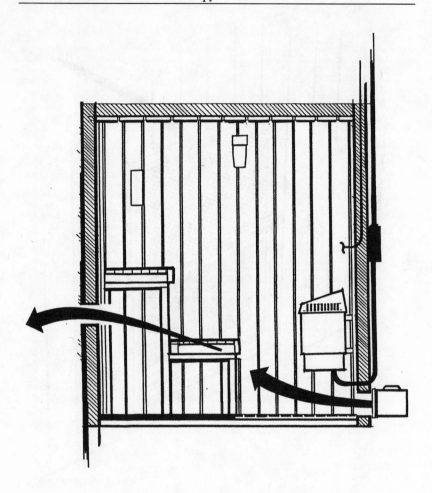

15. Active ventilation: Air filter blowing in

- An air filter unit (such as Allermed's Air Star 5-C™) attached to the side or top of the sauna, to bring in fresh filtered air. An outlet vent must also be provided. (*See Illustration 15.*)
- The air filter unit can be attached to the top or side of the sauna, to pull *out* stale air, and filter it as it enters the exterior room space. An inlet vent must be provided, for incoming air. (*See Illustration 16.*)
- An exhaust fan to pull air from the sauna and blow it into the exterior space, or into duct work which exhausts the sauna air to

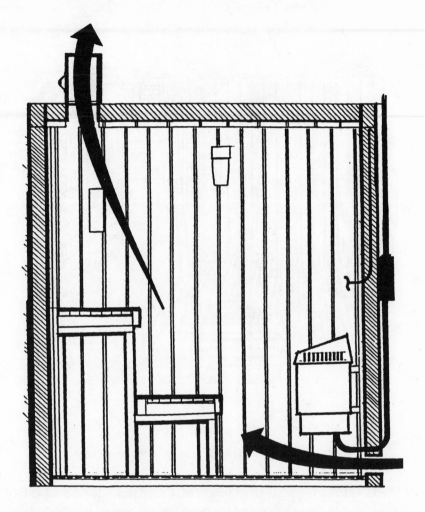

16. Active ventilation: Air filter pulling out

the outdoors. A sheet metal worker can attach a high-temperature blower to a galvanized squirrel-cage, on the exterior of the sauna. This will pull air from the sauna, forcing it to the outdoors via the galvanized duct work. (*See Illustration 17.*)

- An exhaust fan on the exterior of the building (outside), pulling air from the sauna, through the duct work, to the outdoors. (*See Illustration 18.*)

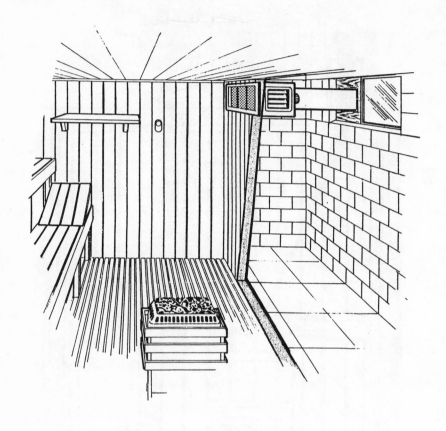

17. Active ventilation: Exhaust fan with squirrel cage

In calculating what size fan you may need, consider the cubic feet of the interior sauna space, and the cubic feet per minute of air exhausted by the particular fan being considered. For example: if the sauna is 6'×6'×6', then the cubic feet is 6 × 6 = 36, 36 × 6 = 216, or 216 cubic feet of interior space. If the blower pulls 82 cfm (cubic feet per minute), then 216 ÷ 82 = 2.63. The total air in the sauna will be exchanged every 2.63 minutes if there is no resistance. The addition of the HEPA (or other) filter will provide resistance, increasing the drag on the fan and decreasing the efficiency. This will increase the time in which the sauna air is exchanged.

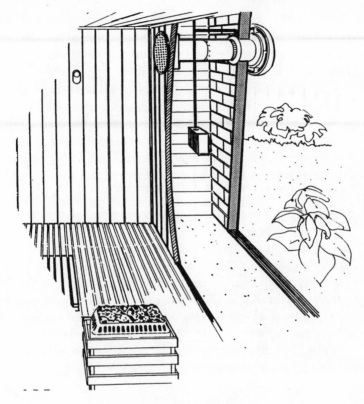

18. Active ventilation: Exhaust fan

Loss of heat through the active ventilation system may concern the energy conscious. However, the air quality inside the sauna can become quite stale without the constant flow of fresh air. Exchanging the air with a fan (or other blower) will make for a more comfortable sauna, with a fresher and more pleasurable air quality. The experience of many has been that the efficiency of the heater is *not* compromised by the addition of a ventilation fan, and the cost to run this system is minimal.

Filtered or Unfiltered Air

The decision on filtering sauna air depends largely on the location of the sauna. The location of the sauna will determine whether or not the incoming air is fresh or polluted, and if the stale sauna air is to be exhausted into the living area or to the outside.

Air can be filtered as it comes in, as it exhausts, or both. Types of filtering material can be HEPA, charcoal, or other chemical filtration media, or a combination, as determined by your particular needs and sensitivities.

A small sauna located in a spare room of your home may be able to pull fresh prefiltered room air in through an open vent in the sauna. Since the stale air will be leaving the sauna and entering the living area, it may be desirable to filter the exhausting air through a charcoal filter.

For a sauna located in a garage, porch or basement, the incoming air may be of questionable quality. In this instance, it may be preferable to filter the air as it enters the unit, and to exhaust stale air to the outdoors.

Benches

There are many designs for sauna benches. The selection of material for the benches is important so that it is safe for skin contact and does not cause abrasion or splinters. Poplar or aspen are well suited for this aspect of sauna construction. Generally, benches are flat, with wooden slats which allow for air flow, and provide enough space for the bathers either to sit or to recline. Bench width is usually 18" to 30" wide for reclining, and 12" to 18" for sitting. Benches have traditionally been arranged in two levels, an upper hotter level and a lower cooler level.

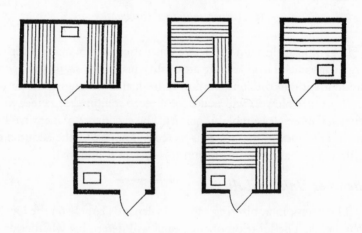

19. Bench arrangements and variations

Benches can be located in a variety of configurations, and at a variety of heights. Some benches are mounted close to the floor, so the feet can rest upon the floor or a duckboard. However, because heat rises, benches are typically mounted closer to the ceiling. Some larger saunas provide both high and low benches, or a narrow 6" step-up bench for access. The lower benches should be about 18" from the floor, and the upper benches no closer than 42" from the ceiling.

The benches should be constructed so that any hardware or nails do not come in contact with the bathers. The benches can be hung from the walls, supported by the floor, or use a combination of both wall and floor support. Benches, although usually built flat, can be built at an angle, or curved to provide a custom-designed environment.

Also available are wood back rests, reclining supports, wood platforms for foot rests, and step stools.

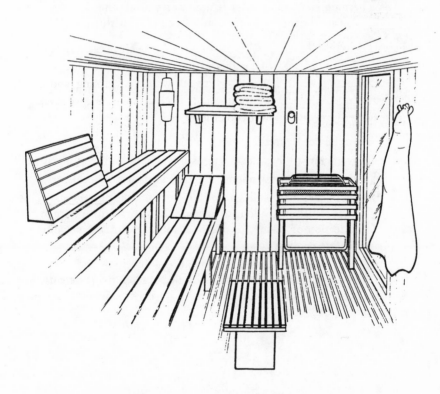

20. Sauna accessories: Back rests, supports, platforms and step stools

Additional Accessories

Many companies offer:

- Wood heater guards to protect bathers from accidental heater burns.
- Extra glass panels in the door or walls, to view the outside, or watch television.
- Latches with ball bullets or rollers that hold the door shut without latching. It is not safe to have a sauna door with a latch that could lock the bather in. Some saunas feature self-closing hinges, which are easy to open with a mere push.
- Wood door handles on both sides of the door.
- Extra windows in the walls of the sauna to allow you to feel less cramped, or provide more light.
- Thermometers, to monitor temperatures inside the sauna. Do not locate the thermometer near the heater, or within 6" of the ceiling.
- Light fixtures, with white or traditional yellow bulbs. Natural or subdued lighting is more restful in a sauna. Light fixtures should not be mounted near the stove, or in the way of bathers. All light switches should be located on the exterior of the sauna.
- Towel racks.
- Bathrobe hooks on the exterior of the sauna.
- Hygrometers to measure the moisture content in the sauna air.
- Intercom, speaker telephone, stereo headphones or speakers.
- Wood buckets with ladles, to ladle water onto the heater rocks. This was traditionally done to increase the sauna temperature by the addition of steam, for one final round of intense perspiration before cooling down.
- Loofahs to scrub the skin, stimulating circulation and increasing perspiration. Traditionally, bundles of birch twigs were used in this fashion. For the chemically sensitive individual this may not be a choice.

7. Some Final Considerations

Taking Responsibility

Take responsibility for your own health care:

- Talk with others, research, ask questions, make telephone calls. No matter what others may say to you, the ultimate responsibility is yours.
- It is your health, your life, your money.
- Go slow. Break the project down into smaller pieces. Do one thing at a time.
- Re-evaluate. Be open to new perspectives, new ideas. Get more information. Do not be afraid to change your mind. If you go slow, you are more likely to achieve success.
- Test your products thoroughly. Retest, if necessary, after receiving new products, new information, or just to compare.
- Detoxification is not just a one-step process. It is a whole way of life. It involves eliminating and reducing toxins in your total environment.

Before Ordering or Purchasing

Before ordering or purchasing any sauna equipment, or deciding to enter a detox center:

- Call the attorney general's office for that state. See if any complaints have been registered about the center or manufacturer you are considering.

- Call the Better Business Bureau for the nearest large town or city. Inquire about the company, its products, its reputation. Take the time to review and study this information, before you make any decisions—it could be vital!

- Get a written contract. Put it all in writing. You can purchase general contract forms at book and stationery stores. It is easier, and better to write your own. List everything to which you and your contractor agreed. Be sure to include the specifications, materials, cost, design specifics, anticipated completion and delivery dates, all included parts, etc. You cannot be too specific. Do not leave anything undocumented. Include a paragraph that reads something to this effect (check with a lawyer in your area):

    We, the undersigned, are entering into this contract in the State of _____. In the event of a disagreement or dispute the matter shall be resolved according to the laws governing the State of _____.

- Make two originals, and have the contractor as well as yourself sign all pages of both copies. This way you each have an original signed copy of the contract.

- Date and record each phone call and transaction, or each correspondence you have with the company or contractor. Get names. Keep a file. Write down the questions, answers, and results from each contact.

- Ask for references. Get the phone numbers of people who have been previous customers or patients. Invest the time to call them. Prepare for these conversations by composing a list of your questions. Listen carefully. Take notes.

- If you are not satisfied with business practices, procedures or outcomes, speak up. If you still are not satisfied, make written complaints to your State's Attorney or Better Business Bureau, or both.

- It is customary for most sauna companies to request 50 percent of the cost when you place your order, and the remaining 50 percent before it is shipped to you. Arranging to pay by C.O.D. gives you the right to refuse the product if it arrives damaged or contaminated during shipping.

- Many companies do not offer the option of C.O.D. and insist on full payment before shipment. If this is the case, use a major credit card. Most major credit card companies offer protection to the consumer, in the event that there is difficulty with the quality of merchandise purchased with the credit card. The advocacy department of the credit company will often carry the credit for the consumer while investigating the dispute. Reasons for dispute can include unauthorized use, the denial of charged merchandise, the refusal of damaged merchandise, or the fraudulent advertising of a product. There is usually no charge to the consumer for this service. Once the dispute is resolved, either payment is refused to the manufacturer of the product, or the charge is assessed to the customer account.

- Before purchasing a major piece of equipment with a credit card, check out the specific policies of the credit card company. Inquire as to the criteria they will accept to advocate a dispute. Some companies require that the consumer attempt to correct the problem, or that the merchandise is returned, and that proof of this is offered, before they will agree to offer advocacy services.

- Whether you purchase your sauna with a credit card, C.O.D., or if you decide to pay with any other method, it is vital that you have signed a contract that covers every aspect of the sauna you believe to be purchasing as well as a clear understanding of when and how it will be shipped, with everything clearly worked out in advance.

About Shipping

There are many things to think about as you plan to have your sauna shipped to you. Do not assume that the manufacturer will just take care of this. Careful arrangements must be made in advance. Consider the following:

- How will the sauna be packaged? In one piece? If so, you will need the dimensions and weight of this package. If the unit comes in several packages, you will need to know the number of boxes to expect, the size and weight of each.

- Will the sauna be protected from contaminants during shipping, and while at the various loading docks along the way? What materials will be used for packaging? Cardboard? Wood? Plastic? Will the packaging cover the sauna completely?

- Most companies have you prepay your shipping charges, usually amounting to hundreds of dollars. Ask for a specific breakdown of what these charges cover.
- Saunas are shipped by huge freight trucks, and may not be the only freight contained on the truck. They are shipped from loading docks, and take many days in transit, as the trucks collect and deposit other freight. These trucks, usually the 16 or 18 wheelers you see on the highway, will probably not be the truck that delivers the sauna to your home.
- Since the larger trucks cannot access many residential neighborhoods, you may have to pay an additional company to get the sauna from the freight company, load it, and bring it to you. The size of your street is important in hiring a truck that can bring the sauna to you.
- Do not assume that the driver of the truck will unload it. Some trucking companies do not permit their drivers to handle the freight. There are union laws, and union truckers abide firmly by them. You may have to hire professional movers to meet the truck, and unload it for you. Some companies, however, will unload it, and leave it at the curb, but their insurance may not permit them to come onto your property.
- Other companies do both moving and hauling, will unload the sauna for you, carry it into your home, and even to the particular spot you desire.
- What are the separate fees involved? Who pays whom? Are personal checks accepted, or will they only accept cash or money orders? Do the drivers expect to receive a tip? Make sure to ask. Know exactly how your sauna will be shipped and delivered. Make sure you hire the right company to do the job.

Rebecca's Story

Rebecca purchased a prefab sauna for several thousand dollars. In addition to the cost of the sauna, several hundred dollars were added for freight. The company required 50 percent of the total cost, as a down payment, prior to assembling the sauna at the factory.

Before the sauna was shipped, the salesperson told her that she could send a check for the remaining 50 percent, or they could ship it

C.O.D. He wanted to advise her, however, that if she chose to pay C.O.D., the trucking company would add 4 to 5 percent of the balance due as "C.O.D. charges." He stressed that if saving money was a factor to her, that she could avoid the C.O.D. charges by paying the balance due before the sauna was shipped.

Of course she wanted to save money! So, she sent in her second and final payment. The sauna was to be delivered within two weeks. A month later, not having heard from the company, she called. The salesman told her the sauna had been shipped three weeks earlier, and suggested she call the trucking company, herself.

The representative at the trucking company told her that the sauna had been sitting at their loading dock for over a week. She explained that she was concerned that the sauna might become contaminated, and that she would like the sauna delivered as soon as possible. The trucking company representative explained that they were not a moving and hauling firm, and that they would bring the truck to her "loading dock," push the boxes to the end of the truck bed, and no further.

She called the sauna salesperson, again, and explained the situation. She stressed that she had paid several hundred dollars for shipping, and that she wanted this problem resolved. He replied that it was her problem, as she had purchased the sauna, and paid for it in full. Ah hah! She haggled with him, stressing the fact that she had ordered and paid for a piece of equipment which she had not received. Because she had paid for it in full, he had no further interest in helping her.

As a last resort, she telephoned the Consumer Protection Agency, which felt that her frustration was justified. However, in the best interests of protecting her sauna from any further contamination, it was important to get it delivered immediately. They advised that she call the trucking firm manager, and be willing to pay an additional fee to work out delivery. Following the delivery of the unit, she could file a complaint with Consumer Protection to recoup her additional expense.

The manager of the trucking company explained that the sauna consisted of eight boxes, several weighing over 200 pounds each, with a total weight of 1,100 pounds. His employees were truck drivers, and not able to lift this type of merchandise. In addition, his huge freight trucks would not be able to navigate her one-lane residential street, nor were they equipped with power tailgate lifts, to unload her sauna to street level. (They customarily back up to loading docks.)

He agreed to subcontract a smaller moving and hauling company to pick up the sauna, load it onto a smaller truck that had a rear tailgate power-lift, and a driver able to unload the 1,100 pounds of boxes into her garage.

Five weeks after she had paid her check, and three weeks later than the anticipated date of delivery, she finally received her sauna, at great additional expense. Then, the carpenter who opened and inspected the boxes found a myriad of problems:

- The protective cartons did not cover the sauna. Large sections of bare wood were exposed, and had been exposed during shipping.
- The plastic heat wrap, promised by the manufacturer to protect the sauna from contaminants, was missing.
- Many pieces and parts to the sauna were missing or back ordered.
- The sauna was not made to the specified dimensions. It was 5" too tall for the intended space.

She now had her sauna. She owned it. She also was the owner of more problems to be solved. Because she had a specific contract with the manufacturer, she was able to pursue a legal remedy, but only at great additional expenditure of time, energy and money.

The entire scenario would have been different if she had used a credit card or paid the extra charges for C.O.D. delivery. The manufacturer might have been more eager to assist in working out the delivery complications. In addition, once the sauna arrived, she could have refused the package when it violated the contract. If at all possible, use a credit card or ship C.O.D.

Arrival

When the assembled or unassembled sauna arrives, expect it to have an odor. Do not expect that any piece of equipment can be introduced into your living space without some degree of upheaval; plan accordingly. Ask for assistance, and plan for this too, as you would plan for any other person entering your living space.

If possible, have the parts, equipment, or sauna delivered to a porch, garage, shed, or separate room where they can be inspected, unpacked, checked and off-gassed. Be creative. Have someone else unpack and check the items against the invoice. Check for damage, missing parts, etc. Remove packaging materials and cardboard boxes as soon as possible. Make any requests or complaints to the company at once.

Do *not* expect to spend time in the same room as the sauna if you are very sensitive. Provide ample ventilation.

Once the Sauna Is Assembled

- Vacuum it
- Wipe it down with plain, tolerated water
- Scrub/wash the heater coils, rocks, and any other removable parts with baking soda and water. Rinse well and air dry. Repeat as necessary for your sensitivities.
- "Bake-out" the sauna. Many manufacturers recommend six to nine hours on "high" to "cure" the sauna. Many MCS people, however, need to extend this time. Three to seven days of running the sauna on "high" for five to eight hours each day, with ample ventilation, is sometimes more helpful. You may need to be at a different location while your sauna is "baking-out."

Before Starting

The day has finally arrived. You have planned, researched, ordered, built, received, assembled, and prepared your sauna. You have baked it out, and are ready to begin. (Do not be surprised if this bake-out time has taken weeks, or even months longer than you expected. Keep at it. In time, the odor and resins of the wood will decrease, especially when the sauna is heated up regularly.)

- Talk with your doctor.
- Go slow. Do not rush in for a one-hour sauna the first day.
- Work up slowly. Start at low temperatures, for short intervals.
- Take plenty of fluids.
- Wear loose clothing.
- Make sure you are taking the necessary supplements, electrolytes, potassium and salt that you need.

• Do not wear sweat clothes in the sauna, they will insulate you.
• According to most sauna programs, 15 to 30 minutes of some form of aerobic exercise is desirable prior to entering the sauna.

Sauna Safety

Saunas are relaxing, invigorating, and easily enjoyed by most persons who are in good health. Heat can be stressful to some individuals. Because the heat in a sauna stimulates the cardiovascular system much in the way exercise does, certain people may need to take shorter saunas and acclimate slowly. In addition, check with your doctor before beginning a sauna program if you are chronically ill, suffering from heart disease, respiratory ailments, diabetes or epilepsy. Patients taking prescription drugs should be aware of any adverse affects. Do not use the sauna if you have been using alcohol or drugs, or if you feel sick, dizzy, nauseated, or experience any cardiac symptoms.[50] Do not exercise or go into the sauna alone. Do not let yourself fall alseep while in the sauna as you run the risk of suffering heat exhaustion or dehydration.

Exercise

Kenneth Cooper states that, "Aerobic exercises refer to those activities that require oxygen for prolonged periods, and place such demands on the body that it is required to improve its capacity to handle oxygen."[51] Aerobic exercise is the recommended type of exercise used in most detoxification programs. Some of the possibilities are running, jumping rope, dancing, rowing, cross-country training machines, or any strenuous exercise that works your heart and lungs. Aerobic exercise:

• Stimulates and causes beneficial changes in the lungs, heart, and vascular system.
• Incites the adrenals to produce hormones that assist in metabolism and excretion.
• Mobilizes fat stores and hastens the excretion of toxins.
• Causes the pituitary gland to release endorphins, which induce a state of well-being, commonly known as "runner's high."[52]

- Increases lung capacity and improves the body's ability to move air into and out of the lungs.
- Improves the strength and efficiency of the heart, improves circulation, and provides a greater protection against heart disease.[53]
- Develops stronger bones.

When exercising:

- Remember that long, slow distances are better than short, fast bursts of energy.
- Exercise sufficiently to keep the body strong and healthy, but not to damage joints and bones.
- Wear comfortable clothing.
- Breathe deeply.
- Have ample ventilation.
- Drink plenty of fluids.[54]

Emotional Climate

The physical and emotional environment in which detoxification takes place is vitally important to its success. Stress and anxiety have an effect on all the organs of the body. Stress can keep the body's detoxification process from working effectively, by slowing peristalsis and digestion, and by causing muscle rigor which affects bowel, bladder, circulatory, and neurological functioning. It is, therefore, important to maintain an atmosphere of relaxation.[55]

You might consider any of the following as an adjunct to your program: stress management, biofeedback, positive imagery, relaxation tapes, massage, meditation, or yoga. Anything geared at keeping the muscles relaxed so the organs within can effectively do their job, may be beneficial. Choose a time for your exercise and sauna when you are not hurried or stressed.

Pay careful attention to the emotional climate you create within the room—this includes lighting, music, furnishings, air quality,

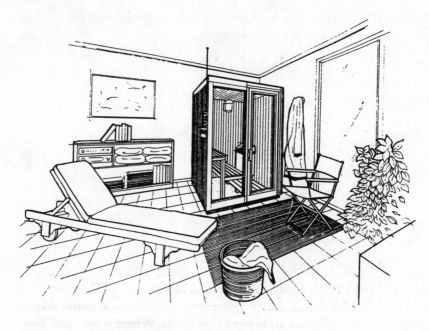

21. A relaxing and inviting sauna environment

temperature, and ventilation. You may want to set up the room so that it is a comfortable, warm, and pleasurable place to enter and a relaxing place to spend your time. You may decide to include some of the following:

- A relaxing chair
- A cot
- Extra towels
- Hooks for robes
- A basket for damp towels and soiled laundry
- A clock
- A timer
- A radio or tape player to provide active music for exercise and relaxing music for saunas. Some people listen to taped meditations, others enjoy talking books. Some prefer silence.

Author's End Note

I have been taking regular saunas for over six years. In these six years I have improved tremendously. I do not spend most of my time in bed or on the couch. I am not running constant fevers, or in constant pain. My food allergies have quieted to a manageable level with careful rotation. On a good day, I can even venture outdoors with oxygen, cotton mask and coverings, and no longer expect to spend three weeks in bed as a consequence.

I am slowly getting better. I know others, who were similarly as severely affected as I, who also seem to be improving. Those who are in the initial and desperately agonizing stages of this dreadful plague, want to know what we are doing to get better. Where is the cure? They will try anything, absolutely anything, to stop the downhill plummet towards total disability.

My personal opinion, based on my own experience and listening to the stories of many others, is that there is no quick fix. There is no sure cure. This is the bad news.

The good news is that time seems to have a lot to do with the immune system's recovery. Time, and a myriad of other variables. These other variables include all the common sense approaches to life that our foremothers and fathers knew—proper rest, proper nutrition, minimal stress, regular exercise, and fresh clean air. These are, however, not easy to obtain in our polluted and frantic society. So, we protect ourselves from the chemicals, eat organic food, filter our air and water, and move to remote locations.

Those who have healed, by and large, have found not one but many modalities which work together to bring a slow healing—a healing with fits and starts, even major setbacks, but nevertheless a climb up out of the mud and muck to a flat and dry place. This flat dry place, this healing, means many different things to different people. Some people recover totally and resume their previous lives and careers. For the most part, however, healing often means the arrival at a place where the illness is controlled with continued vigilance and diligence. Healing, for many, does not mean the end to all physical symptoms of illness. It does not mean that chemical sensitivities disappear, but rather that the individual locates the resources to cope with life, the courage to move forward, and the desire to continue living and finding meaning to life within the structure of each day's activities.

These lucky individuals have often been accompanied by a physician or other medical practitioner who has offered broad-based support, and letters to assist in obtaining job accommodations or benefits. These fortunate patients have benefited from the care of a professional who believed in them, who recognized multiple chemical sensitivity (MCS), who offered patience, expertise, and forbearance over the long, rocky road of their illness.

Those who have healed often seem to exhibit the same qualities as those who heal from other illnesses—a strong sense of responsibility, a fierce will to survive, a determination to solve problems, to fight back, to not give up. They possess a rigorous discipline to get up each day, to soak the beans, carry out the exercise routine, get in that sauna, and just keep moving.

I am aware that there are stories of people who try this or that, took a particular remedy, or who went to a particular place for a period of time and emerged whole and healthy. Many of these cures were expensive, risky, or involved travel and accommodations that were out of reach for me, physically and economically. I opted for a route that gave me a maximum of control over chemical exposures, that was less risky, that had a long history of being tried and true with few side effects, and that was available and affordable. Sauna detoxification therapy filled all of these requirements, and has been a major part of my healing regimen.

I know I will never be completely healed. I will never be the same as I was before my injury, before I became totally disabled with MCS. I know I will never be able to go back to my professional career, or to any type of "normal" life. But the self that has emerged since my disability is a new self. I am more responsible, more self-loving, more socially responsible and aware. The process of deciding to live, involved making other choices and learning to set personal boundaries. At times it has been difficult to keep the boundaries necessary to protect my sleep, food and air-space. In the process, my inner self has become emotionally and psychologically stronger. I have become more committed to a cleaner environment, and to protecting the health of my children and the human race, with which I share this small planet.

The awareness, dedication and discipline involved in a program of total detoxification can revitalize a life. It could also revolutionize the world.

Appendices

The following appendices contain additional information on organizations, suppliers, products, and sources of information mentioned in this text, as well as other resources that may be of interest. These lists are not meant to be exhaustive. For additional information, and information on new products developed for the chemically sensitive, contact the companies, distributors or consultants in the pages that follow. The appendices are:

> Detox Centers
> Sauna Manufacturers
> Distributors
> Consultants
> Product Information
> Periodicals
> Information and Resources
> Organizations
> Suggested Reading List
> Catalog and Mail Order Companies

Detox Centers

The Center for Environmental Medicine
Dr. Allan Lieberman, M.D.
7510 Northforest Drive
North Charlestown, South Carolina 29420
Phone: (803) 572-1600

Environmental Health Center
Dr. William J. Rea, M.D., Director
8345 Walnut Hill Lane, Suite 205
Dallas, Texas 75231
Phone: (214) 368-4123
FAX: (214) 691-8432

HealthMed
Mr. James Woodworth, Administrator
5501 Power Inn Road
Suite 140
Sacramento, California 95820
Phone: (916) 387-8252

Robbins' Environmental Medicine Center
Albert F. Robbins, D.O., M.S.P.H.
400 S. Dixie Highway, Suite 210
Boca Raton, Florida 33432-6023
Phone: (407) 395-3282
Phone: (305) 421-1929

need
20 amp circuit *poplar wood*

most are 15 amp

light *-3 sides glass*
glss *-1 side wood*
wood *whr bch wld be*
-more wood at corners

design w/ platform under a *bench*

$ 2,200
175 - 2 Infrd *special model*
low mag bch rsts

Sauna Manufacturers

40 minutes to heat up

heater 3 amd *radiant bck rst* *2 Infrared heaters*

A mdl w/ skinny heater 110 cnvctn foot rest

Heavenly Heat Saunas
Bob Morgan
1106 Second Street, Suite 162
Encinitas, California 92024
Phone: (619) 942–0401
Phone: (800) MY SAUNA
(800) 697–2862

15- 20¢ per hour

hold 2 adults

The Safe Reading and Computer Box Company
Charlotte Nelson
1158 North Huron
Linwood, Michigan 48634
Phone: (517) 697–3989

light 6'1"
width 3ft
dpth 4ft

1 bench on 4ft
1 platform (hr bench) undr th bnch

has worked w/ autistic kids

Distributors

These companies distribute saunas and other
building products specifically for the environmentally ill.

American Environmental Health Foundation
8345 Walnut Hill Lane
Suite 225
Dallas, Texas 75231–4262
Phone: (800) 428–2343
Phone: (214) 361–9515

E.L. Foust Co., Inc.
P.O. Box 105
Elmhurst, Illinois 60126
Phone: (312) 834–4952

The Living Source
7005 Woodway Drive, Suite 214
Waco, Texas 76712
Phone: (817) 776–4878 (9:00 a.m. to 5:00 p.m. Central Time)
FAX: (817) 776–9392 (order line)
Phone: (800) 662–8787 (24 hour electronic order line)

N.E.E.D.S.
National Ecological and Environmental Delivery System
527 Charles Avenue, 12-A
Syracuse, New York 13209
Phone: (315) 488–6312
Phone: (800) 634–1380

Nigra Enterprises
5699 Kanan Road
Agoura, California 91301
Phone: (818) 889–6877

Consultants

The following consultants offer resources and information to those with MCS.

Clarity House
Limited Liability Company
Earle Meek, President
45 Chipmunk Hill
Berkeley Springs, West Virginia 25411
Phone: (304) 258-9029
>*Provides information on housing accessibility, land searches, building materials, and the design and construction of safe housing for the chemically sensitive*

Environmental Education and Health Services, Inc.
Mary Oetzel
P.O. Box 92004
Austin, Texas 78709-2004
Phone: (512) 288-2369
>*Provides information, referrals and resources for building, job accessibility, renovations and safe construction techniques for homes and schools*

Environmental Health Center
Carolyn Gorman, M.A. Health Education
8345 Walnut Hill Lane
Suite 205
Dallas, Texas 75231
Phone: (214) 337-5146
>*Consultations about a wide variety of topics concerning the chemically sensitive*

Healthy Buildings Associates
Dan Morris
1932 First Avenue, #515
Seattle, Washington 98101
Phone: (206) 448–9135
Offers telephone or on-site consultations on all aspects of safe housing

Healthy House Institute
John Bower
430 N. Sewell Road
Bloomington, Indiana 47408
Phone: (812) 332–5073
Information, videos and books on the design and construction of healthy houses

Nigra Enterprises
Jim Nigra
5699 Kanan Road
Agoura, California 91301-3328
Phone: (818) 889-6877
Information on building, accessibility, renovations, and a wide variety of products for environmental purification

Product Information

*The following products may be useful to the chemically
sensitive in building saunas or other construction projects.*

AFM
American Formulating and Manufacturing, Inc.
Sam Goldberg, President
Suite 700
350 West Ash Street
San Diego, California 92101
Phone: (619) 239–0321
> *Manufacturers of an entire line of less-toxic personal and building
> supplies, compounded specifically for the chemically sensitive*

Air Krete
Palmer Industries Inc.
Doug Carmen, President
Suite 700
10611 Old Annapolis Road
Frederick, Maryland 21701
Phone: (301) 898–7848
> *Manufacturers and distributors of nontoxic pumped-in cementitious foam
> insulation*

AirStar 5-C
AllerMed
Boyd Hager, President
31 Steel Road
Wylie, Texas 75098
Phone: (214) 442–4898
> *Manufacturers of various sizes of air filters, with various filtration media
> for a variety of uses and situations*

Autoclaved Aerated Concrete
Hebel U.S.A.
P.O. Box 767220
Roswell, Georgia 30076
Phone: (404) 552–8665
> *A line of building products that are durable, easy to work with, nontoxic, low maintenance, and fire, wind and pest resistant*

Cerablanket
Thermal Ceramics Inc.
Rich Waugh, Manager of Marketing and Communications
P.O. Box 923
Augusta, Georgia 30903
Phone: (800) KAO WOOL
Phone: (706) 796–4252
> *Specialize in the manufacture of insulating refractories*

Ceramic Radiant Heater Corporation
P.O. Box 60
Greenport, New York 11944
Phone: (800) 331–6408
> *Makers of stainless steel radiant heaters designed specifically for the environmentally ill*

Class A Blowing Insulation
Knauf Fiber Glass
240 Elizabeth Street
Shelbyville, Indiana 46171
Phone: (317) 398–4434
> *Makers of various insulating materials*

Dennyfoil
Denny Corporation
Route 4
Caldwell, Ohio 43724
Phone: (619) 732–5665
> *Manufacturers of various types of aluminum reflective vapor barrier insulation*

Foil-Ray
Elnathan Thermal 'R' Systems
Division of Elnathan Resources Company
North Lee Road
P.O. Box 7528
Odessa, Texas 79760
Phone: (915) 337–5581
*Master dealer/distributor of reflective insulation and reflective barrier
materials*

Formaldehye-Free Medium Density Fiberboard (MDF)
Medite Corporation
P.O. Box 4040
Medford, Oregon 97501
Phone: (503) 779–9596
Phone: (503) 773–2522
Phone: (800) 676–3339
A variety of pressed-wood products that do not contain formaldehyde

Fresh Air Ventilation Systems
DEC International Inc.
Therma-Stor Products Group
1919 S. Stoughton Rd.
P.O. Box 8050
Madison, Wisconsin 53708
Phone: (608) 222–3484
A variety of ventilation systems for small areas or entire buildings

G.E. Silicones
General Electric Company
260 Hudson River Rd.
Mail Stop 80-38
Waterford, New York 12188
Phone: (800) 505–7355
*A line of silicone products, including 100% pure silicone acetic-acid cured
caulking without dyes*

Greenwood Cotton Insulation
Greenwood Cotton Insulation Products, Inc.
Division of Greenwood Mills, Inc.
P.O. Box 1017
Greenwood, South Carolina 29648
Phone: (800) 546–1332
Manufacturers of R11, R13, R19 and R30 cotton insulation with Kraft paper facing

InsulSafe III
CertainTeed Corporation
Tom Newton, Communications
P.O. Box 860
Valley Forge, Pennsylvania 19482
Phone: (800) 441–9850
Phone: (610) 341–7739
Makers of various types of insulating materials

Landmark Logworks
3489 Landmark Rd.
The Plains, Virginia 22171
Phone: (540) 687–4124
A source for hard-to-locate untreated lumber

Miller Paint Company Inc.
317 SE Grand Avenue
Portland, Oregon 97214
Phone: (503) 233–4491
Paints without biocides and other noxious ingredients

Old Fashioned Milk Paint Co.
P.O. Box 222
436 Main Street
Groton, Massachusetts 01450
Phone: (508) 448–6336
Powdered paints made from milk, with safer dyes in a variety of colors and textures

Palmer Bedding Company
9310 Keystone St.
Philadelphia, Pennsylvania 19114
Phone: (215) 335–0400
> *Custom-made mattresses, cushions, and other upholstery needs, from nontoxic and natural sources*

Polyken
The Kendall Company
15 Hampshire Street
Mansfield, Massachusetts 02048
Phone: (800) 248–7659
Makers of various foil tapes and aluminum foil products

High Standard, Inc.
P.O. Box 446
Dublin, New Hampshire 03444
Phone: (800) 358–8018
> *Manufacturers of various architectural panel products including lightweight porcelain on steel panels, in a variety of colors, widths and thicknesses.*

Reflectix, Inc.
P.O. Box 108
Markleville, Indiana 46056
Phone: (800) 233–3645
Phone: (317) 533–4332
> *Manufacturers of reflective bubble insulation*

Right-On Crystal Shield
Right-On Crystal Aire
Pace Chem Industries, Inc.
779 South La Grange Avenue
Newberry Park, California 91320
Phone: (805) 499–2911
> *Makers of less-toxic sealants*

Stainless Steel Foil
Alpine Industries
P.O. Box 277
Mount Shasta, CA 96067
Phone: (916) 926–2460
Provide rolls of stainless steel foil which is tough and durable, but malleable for a variety of uses

Thermoply
Simplex Products Division
P.O. Box 10
Adrian, Michigan 49221
Foil-backed insulated wall sheathing

Periodicals

*These publications provide information vital
to those living with chemically induced illnesses*

The Delicate Balance
Mary Lamielle, Editor
1100 Rural Avenue
Voorhees, New Jersey 08043
Phone: (609) 429-5358
Prodigy: WJRD37A
Internet: WJRD37A@PRODIGY.COM
> *Quarterly publication of the National Center for Environmental Health
> Strategies*

The Green Guide
Mindy Pennybacker, Editor
40 West 20th Street
New York, New York 10011
Phone: (888) ECO-INFO
> *Newsletter of Mothers and Others for a Liveable Planet, published 15
> times a year*

The Human Ecologist
Diane C. Thomas, Editor
P.O. Box 49126
Atlanta, Georgia 30359-1126
Phone: (404) 248-1898
> *Quarterly publication of the Human Ecology Action League*

The New Reactor
P.O. Box 1155
Larkspur, California 94977
> *Newsletter of the Environmental Health Network*

Our Toxic Times
Cynthia Wilson, Editor
P.O. Box 301
White Sulphur Springs, Montana 59645
Phone: (406) 547–2255
  Monthly publication of the Chemical Injury Information Network

Pesticides and You
Jay Feldman, Editor and Publisher
701 E Street, SE
Washington, D.C. 20003
Phone: (202) 543–5450
FAX: (202) 543–4791
Email: ncamp@igc.apc.org
  Quarterly publication of the National Coalition Against the Misuse of Pesticides

Solutions
James C. Moore, Editor
New York Coalition for Alternatives to Pesticides
353 Hamilton Street
Albany, New York 12210–1709
Phone: (518) 426–8246
  A quarterly news magazine published by the New York Coalition for Alternatives to Pesticides

Information and Resources

See also the following appendix, Organizations.

Chemical Injury Information Network
Cynthia Wilson
P.O. Box 301
White Sulphur Springs, Montana 59645
Phone: (406) 547–2255
> *Provides support and information about news items, legislation and a wide range of topics of interest to those injured by chemical exposure*

E.A.R.N.
Environmental Access Research Network
Cindy Duehring
P.O. Box 426
Williston, North Dakota 58802–0426
Phone: (701) 859–6363 (Monday–Wednesday, 8:00 a.m. to 1:00 p.m., Central Time)
> *Provides research on medical topics, data based computer searches, articles and investigative searches on topics of interest to those injured by chemicals or those seeking specific information on chemical injury and related health issues*

Housing for the Environmentally Hypersensitive
Canadian Housing Study
Prepared in 1990 by:
Drerup Armstrong Limited
P.O. Box 130
Carp, Ontario, Canada K0A 1L0
Phone: (613) 836–1494
> *A wealth of information on many facets of building for the environmentally ill*

M.C.S. Referral & Resources
Albert Donnay, MHS, Project Director
2326 Pickwick Road
Baltimore, Maryland 21207–6631
Phone: (410) 448–3319
> *Provides support and advocacy for patients desiring education, literature, referrals, research services, diagnosis, treatment, prevention, and information on accommodations*

National Pesticide Telecommunications Network
Oregon State University
Department of Agricultural Chemistry
Weniger Hall, Room 333
Corvallis, Oregon 97331–6502
Phone: (800) 858–PEST
Phone: (800) 858–7378
> *Information into toxicity data and other information about specific pesticides*

The Neurotoxicity Advice and Information Line
36 Alondra Road
Santa Fe, New Mexico 87505
Phone: (505) 466–1100
> *Provides information and referral service on neurotoxic effects of chemical injury*

Office of the Americans with Disabilities Act
Civil Rights Division
U.S. Department of Justice
Box 66118
Washington, D.C. 20035
Phone: (202) 514–0301
Phone: (202) 514–0381
Phone: (202) 514–0383 (TDD)
> *Provides copies of the law, and other pertinent information related to the ADA*

Organizations

*Many of these organizations are helpful to those
seeking information about chemical injury or illness, and related
issues. In addition, many of these organizations produce their own
newsletters. See also the previous appendix, Information and Resources.*

American Academy of Environmental Medicine
4510 W 89th Street
Prairie Village, Kansas 66207
Phone: (913) 642–6062

American Association for Retired Persons
Health Advocacy
601 E Street, N.W.
Washington, D.C. 20049
Phone: (202) 434–2277

American Chronic Pain Association
P.O. Box 850
Rocklin, California 95677
Phone: (916) 632–0922

American Silicone Implant Survivors
1288 Cork Elm Drive
Kirkwood, Missouri 63122
Phone: (314) 821–0115

Arthritis Foundation
P.O. Box 19000
Atlanta, Georgia 30326
Phone: (800) 283–7800

The Bio-Integral Resource Center
P.O. Box 7414
Berkeley, California 94707
Phone: (510) 524–2567

Candida and Dysbiosis Information Foundation
P.O. Drawer JF
College Station, Texas 77841
Phone: (409) 694–8687

Candida Research Foundation
1638 B Street
Hayward, California 94541
Phone: (510) 582–2179

Center for Rehabilitation Science
Louisiana Tech University
Michael Shipp
P.O. Box 3185
Ruston, Louisiana 71272–0001
Phone: (318) 257–4562

Centers for Disease Control
1600 Clifton Road NE
Atlanta, Georgia 30333
Phone: (404) 639–3311

The CFIDS Association, Inc.
P.O. Box 220398
Charlotte, North Carolina 28222–0398
Phone: (800) 442–3437
Phone: (704) 362–2343

CFIDS Foundation
965 Mission Street #425
San Francisco, California 94103
Phone: (415) 882–9986

Chemical Injury Research Foundation
3639 North Pearl Street
Tacoma, Washington 98407

Chemically Injured Federal Workers
17402 6th Avenue SW
Seattle, Washington 98166–3722
Phone: (206) 244–9345

Children Afflicted by Toxic Substances (C.A.T.S.)
60 Oscer Avenue #1
Hauppauge, New York 11788
Phone: (800) CATS–199

Clearinghouse on Disability Information
Office of Special Education and Rehabilitation Services
U.S. Department of Education
Room 3132, Switzer Building
Washington, D.C. 20202

Coalition of Silicone Survivors
P.O. Box 129
Broomfield, Colorado 80038–0129
Phone: (303) 469–8242

Dental Amalgam Mercury Syndrome (D.A.M.S.)
6025 Osuna Road N.E. #B
Albuquerque, New Mexico 87109–2523
Phone: (505) 888–0111

Desert Storm Veterans Coalition
P.O. Box 2313
Hewitt, Texas 76643–2313
Phone: (800) 307–1330
Phone: (817) 666–2175

Environmental Health Network
Great Bridge Station, P.O. Box 16267
Chesapeake, Virginia 23328–6267
Phone: (804) 424–1162

Environmental Protection Agency, U.S. (E.P.A.)
Public Information Center, PM-211B
401 M Street, S.W.
Washington, D.C. 20460
Phone: (202) 260–2080

Environmental Research Foundation
P.O. Box 5036
Annapolis, Maryland 21403–7036
Phone: (253) 1584

Fibromyalgia Network
P.O. Box 31750
Tucson, Arizona 85751–1750
Phone: (602) 290–5508

or

5700 Stockdale Highway #100
Bakersfield, California 93309
Phone: (805) 631–1950

Foundation for Advancements in Science and Education (FASE)
4801 Wilshire Boulevard
Park Mile Plaza
Los Angeles, California 90010
Phone: (213) 937–9911

Foundation for Environmental Health Research
1760 East River Road #139A
Tucson, Arizona 85718–5876
Phone: (602) 577–5225

Foundation for Toxic Free Dentistry
P.O. Box 608010
Orlando, Florida 32860–0818

Human Ecology Action League (HEAL)
P.O. Box 49126
Atlanta, Georgia 30359
Phone: (404) 248–1898

Independent Agent Orange Network
6806 36th Avenue SE
Olympia, Washington 98503

Institute for Safe Living for the Chemically Injured
1038 Woodlawn
Grand Haven, Michigan 49417

International Resource Center for the Chemically Disabled and
    Immune Compromised
9736 West Reeves Court
Franklin Park, Illinois 60131
Phone: (708) 678–5934

Mothers and Others for a Liveable Planet
40 West 20th Street
New York, New York 10011

National Center for Environmental Health Strategies (NCEHS)
Mary Lamielle, President
1100 Rural Avenue
Voorhees, New Jersey 08043
Phone: (609) 429–5358

National Coalition Against the Misuse of Pesticides (NCAMP)
701 E Street SE #200
Washington, DC 20003
Phone: (202) 543–5450

National Institute for Occupational Safety and Health (NIOSH)
Building 1, Room 3106
1600 Clifton Road, N.E.
Atlanta, Georgia 30333
Phone: (404) 331–2396

   or

4676 Columbia Parkway
Cincinnati, Ohio 45226
Phone: (800) 35NIOSH
Phone: (513) 533–8236

National Institute of Allergy and Infectious Disease (NIAID)
Office of Communications
9000 Rockville Pike
Building 31, Room 7A32
Bethesda, Maryland 20892
Phone: (301) 496–5717

National Institute of Environmental Health Sciences (NIEHS)
Public Affairs Office
P.O. Box 12233
Research Triangle Park, North Carolina 27709
Phone: (919) 541–3345

National Institute of Neurological Disorders and Stroke
National Institutes of Health
Bethesda, Maryland 20892–2540
Phone: (301) 496–5751

National Organization for Rare Disorders
P.O. Box 8923
New Fairfield, Connecticut 06812
Phone: (203) 746–6518

**National Organization of Legal Advocates for the Environmentally
    Injured**
P.O. Box 29507
Atlanta, Georgia 30329
Phone: (404) 264–4445

National Research Council (NRC)
National Academy of Sciences
2101 Constitution Avenue, N.W.
Washington, D.C. 20418
Phone: (202) 334–2000

Occupational Safety and Health Administration (OSHA)
U.S. Department of Labor
200 Constitution Avenue, N.W.
Room N-3647
Washington, D.C. 20210
Phone: (202) 523–8148

Rachel Carson Council, Inc.
8940 Jones Mill Road
Chevy Chase, Maryland 20815
Phone: (301) 652–1877
Email: rccouncil@col.com

Rehabilitation Engineering Society of North America
John Greene
1101 Connecticut Avenue, Suite 700
Washington, D.C. 20036
Phone: (202) 857–1199

Share Care and Prayer Ministry, Inc.
P.O. Box 2080
Frazier Park, California 93225

Victims of Fiberglass
P.O. Box 162646
Sacramento, California 95816–2646
Phone: (916) 452–2834

Victims of Isocyanates
HC 61 Box 167
Deerwood, Minnesota 56444
Phone: (218) 546–6446

Well Spouse Foundation
P.O. Box 28876
San Diego, California 92198

Suggested Reading List for Coping with the Emotional Side of Chronic Illness

Beisser, Arnold R. *Flying Without Wings: Personal Reflections on Being Disabled*. New York: Doubleday, 1989. A personal and vivid account of a man's attempt to find meaning in his life following the onset of chronic illness.

Burns, David D. *The Feeling Good Handbook*. New York: A Plume Book, Penguin, 1989. A sequel to his previous book, *Feeling Good: The New Mood Therapy*, continues to give information and techniques to cope with conflict, fears and anxiety.

Cousins, Norman. *Anatomy of an Illness as Perceived by the Patient: Reflections on Healing and Regeneration*. New York: Bantam Books, 1979. A personal account of a man's ability to use humor to help his body heal from crippling illness.

Duff, Kat. *The Alchemy of Illness*. New York: Pantheon Books, 1993. The journey of a woman coping with chronic fatigue syndrome, and her attempt to find meaning in the face of illness.

Halperin, Deanne H. *Chronic Illness: Dealing with Fear*. Minnesota: Hazelden, 1988. A short pamphlet-type book covering the psychological stages of coming to terms with chronic illness by the use of acceptance, trust and faith.

Hay, Louise L. *Life, Reflections on Your Journey*. Carson, California: Hay House, 1995. Reflections about the journey of life and the challenges, fears and obstacles that are encountered.

_____. *You Can Heal Your Life*. Santa Monica, California: Hay House, 1984. A guide to healing through imagery.

Lewis, Kathleen. *Successful Living with Chronic Illness*. Wayne, New Jersey: Avery Publishing Group, 1985. A concise exploration of the psychological aspects of chronic illness.

McWilliams, Peter and John-Roger. *You Can't Afford the Luxury of a Negative Thought*. Los Angeles: Prelude Press, 1988. The power of positive thinking and avoiding negative thinking to help promote healing.

Peck, M. Scott, M.D. *Further Along the Road Less Traveled: The Unending Journey Toward Spiritual Growth*. New York: Simon and Schuster, 1993. A continuation of his previous book, with expanded lecture material emphasizing personal growth.

_____. *The Road Less Traveled: A New Psychology of Love, Traditional Values and Spiritual Growth*. New York: Simon and Schuster, 1978. Suggestions about coping with changes, loss, grief and suffering through self understanding.

Baumer Permut, Joanna. *Embracing the Wolf: A Lupus Victim and Her Family Learn to Live with Chronic Disease*. A personal account of the social and emotional effects of living with chronic illness.

Pitzele, Sefra Kobrin. *We Are Not Alone: Learning to Live with Chronic Illness*. New York: Workman Publishing Co., 1985, 1986. An up-beat and practical guide on the emotional side of chronic illness.

Siegel, Bernie S., M.D. *Love, Medicine and Miracles: Lessons Learned about Self-Healing from a Surgeon's Experience with Exceptional Patients*. Harper & Row, New York, 1986. A doctor's rendition of his encounters with the miraculous healing and recovery of certain patients, and their similarities in approaching their illnesses.

Solomon, Marion F., Ph.D. *Lean on Me: The Power of Positive Dependency in Intimate Relationships*. New York: Simon and Schuster, 1994. A discussion of independence and interdependence in relationships.

Stearns, Ann Kaiser. *Living Through Personal Crisis*. New York: Ballantine Books, 1984. Case stories of personal losses and advice on coping with these experiences and healing from the grief.

Strong, Maggie. *Mainstay: For the Well Spouse of the Chronically Ill.* Penguin Books, 1988. A personal account of the emotional and practical side of being related to a person with chronic illness.

Weil, Andrew, M.D. *Spontaneous Healing.* New York: Alfred A. Knopf, 1995. A presentation of the phenomenon of spontaneous healing, including the participation of environmental factors in the body's recovery.

Catalog and
Mail Order Companies

The following catalogs and mail order companies offer items of
special interest to those living with multiple chemical sensitivities.

Allergy Alternative
440 Godfrey Drive
Windsor, California 95492
Phone: (800) 838–1514
   Skin care products, supplements, household products, air cleaners, water purifiers

American Environmental Health Foundation
8345 Walnut Hill Lane
Suite 225
Dallas, Texas 75231–4262
Phone: (800) 428–2343
Phone: (214) 361–9515
   Air filters, bedding, books, clothing, furniture, medical supplies, pet
   supplies, personal hygiene, cleaning supplies, saunas, heaters, reading
   boxes, water filtration systems, etc.

Back to Basics Soft-Wear, Inc.
P.O. Box 432
Bahama, North Carolina 27503–0432
Phone: (919) 477–5669
FAX: (919) 477–6476
   Women's cotton undergarments

The Cotton Place
P.O. Box 7715
Waco, Texas 76714
Phone: (817) 751–7730
Order Line: (800) 451–8866
   Cotton clothing, fabrics, bedding, household items and personal care products

The Culpepper Company
P.O. Box 266
Clinton, Louisiana 70722
Phone: (504) 683–4198
> *Bedding, building items, kitchen items, supplements, water purification systems, clothing, and assorted items*

Deva Lifewear
110 1st Avenue West
P.O. Box 6A
Westhope, North Dakota 58793–0266
Phone: (800) 222–8024
> *Cotton clothing for men and women*

Environmentally Sound Products, Inc.
1703 East Joppa Road
Baltimore, Maryland 21234
Phone: (410) 661–3500
Phone: (800) 886–5432
> *Environmental products*

Fisher Henney Natural's
P.O. Box 590336
San Francisco, California 94159
Phone: (800) 343–6639
> *Women's cotton and natural fiber dresses and suits*

E.L. Foust, Inc.
P.O. Box 105
Elmhurst, Illinois 60126
Phone: (800) 225–9549
> *Air filters, water purification systems and miscellaneous items*

Furnature Inc.
319 Washington Street
Brighton, Massachusetts 02135
Phone: (617) 782–3939
> *Formaldehyde-free furniture*

Heart of Vermont
P.O. Box 612
Barre, Vermont 05641
Phone (800) 639–4123
Organic bedding and associated items

Janice's
198 Route 46
Budd Lake, New Jersey 07828
Phone: (800) JANICES
Cotton clothing, bedding, custom made mattresses and box springs,
fabrics, household and personal items

Lehman's Non-Electric Catalogue
One Lehman Circle
P.O. Box 41
Kidron, Ohio 44636
Phone: (216) 857–5757
A wide variety of non-electric utilitarian household and other hard-to-
find items

The Living Source
P.O. Box 20155
Waco, Texas 76702
Phone: (817) 776–4878
Order Line: (800) 662–8787
Products for the chemically sensitive, including personal products,
cosmetics, heaters, air and water filtration systems, bedding, books,
supplements, pet care and more

Natural Baby Company Inc.
816 Sylvia Street 800B/S
Trenton, New Jersey 08628–3299
Phone: (800) 388–2229
Natural baby clothing and related items

The Natural Choice
Eco Design Company
1365 Rufina Circle
Santa Fe, New Mexico 87505
Phone: (800) 621–2591
Paints, shoe care, floor care, wood finishes and other healthy home products

Natural Selections
872 South Milwaukee Avenue #124
Libertyville, Illinois 60048
Phone: (847) 367–8271
> *A variety of environmental products including cleaning products, dietary supplements, air and water filtration systems*

N.E.E.D.S.
National Ecological and Environmental Delivery System
527 Charles Avenue 12A
Syracuse, New York 13209
Phone: (800) 634–1380
> *Supplements, domestics, cosmetics, air and water purifiers, books*

Real Goods
555 Leslie Street
Ukiah, California 95482–5576
Phone: (800) 762–7325
> *Household items, paper products, furniture, clothing, garden supplies and miscellaneous environmental products*

Reflections Organic Inc.
214 North Lewis Street
Route 1, Box 348
Trinity, Texas 75862–9407
Phone: (800) 852–9273
> *Organically grown cotton clothing for men and women*

Seventh Generation
One Mill Street
Box A26
Burlington, Vermont 05401–1530
Phone: (800) 456–1177
> *Household items, bedding, disposable paper products, clothing, garden supplies, and other miscellaneous environmental products*

The Vermont Country Store
P.O. Box 3000
Manchester Center, Vermont 05255–3000
Phone: (802) 362–2400
> *Cotton clothing and hard-to-find household and personal items*

Walnut Acres
Organic Farms
Penns Creek, Pennsylvania 17862
Phone: (800) 433-3998
Organically grown foods

Winter Silks
2700 Laura Lane
P.O. Box 620130
Middleton, Wisconsin 53562
Phone: (800) 648-7455
Phone: (800) 621-3229
Men and women's silk clothing

References

1. Nicholas Ashford and Claudia Miller, *Chemical Exposures: Low Levels and High Stakes* (New York: Van Nostrand Reinhold, 1991) 10.

2. David Root and Joan Anderson, "Reducing Toxic Body Burdens Advancing in Innovative Technique," *Occupational Health and Safety Digest* 2, 4 (April 1986).

3. Ashford and Miller, *Chemical Exposures*, 8, 51.

4. Gunner Heuser, M.D., "Diagnotic Markers in Clinical Immunotoxicology and Neurotoxicology," *Journal of Occupational Medicine and Toxicology* 1, 4 (1992).

5. William J. Meggs, M.D. and Crawford H. Cleveland, Jr., M.D., "Rhinolaryngoscopic Examination of Patients with the Multiple Chemical Sensitivity Syndrome," *Archives of Environmental Health* 48, 1 (1993) 14–18.

6. Stephen A. Schacker, M.D., "A Triune Brain Model of MCS Syndrome," *Our Toxic Times* 4, 7 (1993) 1–3.

7. Thomas J. Callendar, Lisa Morrow, Kodanullar Subramanian, Dan Duhon, and Mona Ristovv, "Three-Dimensional Brain Metabolic Imaging in Patients with Toxic Encephalopathy," *Environmental Research* 60 (1993) 295–319.

8. Gordon P. Baker, M.D., "Porphyria and MCS Overlap Symptoms," *Our Toxic Times*, 5, 8 (1994) 1–5.

9. Stephen Barron, *Survey of the Medical Impact on Environmentally Hypersensitive People of a Change in Habitat* (Ottawa: Canada Mortgage and Housing Corporation, 1990) 46–47.

10. Barron, *Survey of the Medical Impact*, 58.

11. Leonard A. Jason, Ph.D., and Trina Davis, "M.C.S. Treatment Evaluation Survey of 305 Participants," DePaul University, undated.

12. Susan Wharton and Paul Spring, *Spas, Hot Tubs, and Home Saunas* (Menlo Park, Calif.: Lane Publishing Co., 1989) 67.

13. Jacqueline Krohn, M.D., *The Whole Way to Allergy Relief and Prevention, a Doctor's Complete Guide to Treatment and Self-Care* (Point Roberts, Washington: Hartley and Marks, Inc., 1991) 255–257.

14. Richard D. Swartz, M.D., and Frederick R. Sidell, M.D., "Effects of Heat and Exercise on the Elimination of Pralidoxime in Man," Clinical Investigation

Section, Biomedical Laboratory, Edgewood Arsenal, Maryland, paper presented in part at the Federation of American Societies for Experimental Biology Meeting, American Society for Pharmacology and Experimental Therapeutics Section, Atlantic City, N.J., April 10, 1972.

15. L. Ron Hubbard, *Clear Body: Clear Mind—The Effective Purification Program* (Los Angeles: Bridge Publications, 1990) vii–27.

16. James R. Cohn, M.S., and Edward A. Emmett, M.B., B.S., M.S., F.R.A.C.P., "The Excretion of Trace Metals in Human Sweat," *Annals of Clinical and Laboratory Science* 8, 4 (1978) 270–274.

17. Edwin Chen, *PBB: An American Tragedy* (Englewood Cliffs: Prentice-Hall, Inc., 1979) xi.

18. Mary S. Wolff, H.A. Anderson, K.D. Rosenman, and I.J. Selikoff, "Equilibrium of Polybrominated Biphenyl (PBB) Residues in Serum and Fat of Michigan Residents," *Bulletin of Environmental Contamination and Toxicology* 21, 6 (1979) 775–781.

19. Mary S. Wolff, Ph.D., Henry A. Anderson, M.D., Irving J. Selikoff, M.D., "Human Tissue Burdens of Halogenated Aromatic Chemicals in Michigan," *Journal of the American Medical Association* 247, 15 (April 16, 1982) 2112–2116.

20. D.W. Schnare, G. Denk, M. Shields, S. Brunton, "Evaluation of a Detoxification Regimen for Fat Stored Xenobiotics," *Medical Hypotheses* 9 (1982) 265–282.

21. Dan Christian Roehm, "Effects of a Program of Sauna Baths and Megavitamins on Adipose DDE and PCB's and on Clearing of Symptoms of Agent Orange (Dioxin) Toxicity," *Clinical Research* 31, 2 (1983) 243A.

22. Robert B. Amidon, "Chemical Hazards in Law Enforcement," *Journal of California Law Enforcement* 18, 3 (Summer 1984) 27–30.

23. David W. Schnare, Max Ben, and Megan G. Shields, "Body Burden Reductions of PCBs, PBBs and Chlorinated Pesticides in Human Subjects," *Ambio* 13, 5-6 (1984) 378–380.

24. David E. Root, M.D., M.P.H., and Gerald T. Lionelli, B.S., "Excretion of a Lipophilic Toxicant Through the Sebaceous Glands: A Case Report," *Journal of Toxicology* 6, 1 (1987) 13–17.

25. Kaye H. Kilburn, M.D., Raphael H. Warsaw, Megan G. Shields, M.D., "Neurobehavioral Dysfunction in Firemen Exposed to Polychlorinated Biphenyls (PCBs): Possible Improvement after Detoxification," *Archives of Environmental Health* 44, 6 (1989b) 345–350.

26. Kaye H. Kilburn, M.D., "Is the Human Nervous System Most Sensitive to Environmental Toxins?" *Archives of Environmental Health* 44, 6 (Nov./Dec. 1989) 343–344.

27. Ziga Tretjak, Shelley Beckman, Ana Tretjak, Charles Gunnerson, "Occupational, Environmental, and Public Health in Semic: A Case Study of Polychlorinated Biphenyl (PCB) Pollution," reprinted from Post-Audits of Environmental

Programs and Projects Proceedings, Environmental Impact Analysis Research Council, ASCE, New Orleans (October 11, 1989) 57–72.

28. David E. Root, M.D., M.P.H., "Reducing Toxic Body Burdens Advancing in Innovative Technique," *Occupational Health and Safety News Digest* 2, 4 (April 1986).

29. Phyllis Saifer and Merla Zellerback, *Detox* (New York: Ballantine Books, 1984) 28.

30. Jean Marbella, "How We Sweat," *Baltimore Sun*, April 28, 1992.

31. Grace Ziem, "Multiple Chemical Sensitivity: Treatment and Follow-up with Avoidance and Control of Chemical Exposures," *Toxicology and Industrial Health* 8 (1992) 73.

32. Ziem, "Multiple Chemical Sensitivity," 73.

33. Ashford and Miller, *Chemical Exposures*, 67–68.

34. Saifer and Zellerback, *Detox*, 27.

35. Debra Lynn Dadd, *Non-Toxic, Natural, and Earthwise* (Los Angeles: Jeremy P. Tarcher, Inc., 1990) 77.

36. Dadd, *Non-Toxic*, 81.

37. Ashford and Miller, *Chemical Exposures*, 135–136.

38. L. Ron Hubbard Library, *Purification Rundown Delivery Manual* (Los Angeles: Bridge Publications, 1990).

39. Schnare, D.W., G. Denk, M. Shields, M.D., and S. Brunton, "Evaluation of a Detoxification Regimen for Fat Stored Xenobiotics," *Medical Hypotheses* 9 (1982) 265–282.

40. Hubbard, *Clear Body: Clear Mind*, 43–59.

41. *Ibid.* 117–130.

42. Environmental Health Center—Dallas, "Physical Therapy Program," photocopy, 1992.

43. *Ibid.*

44. Carolyn Gorman, Environmental Health Center—Dallas, letter to author, November 22, 1991.

45. Bob Morgan, Heavenly Heat Sauna, Encinitas, California, telephone conversation with author, January, 1992.

46. Kathryn Metzger, "Glass Greenhouse Becomes Sauna," *The Human Ecologist* 49 (Summer 1991) 16.

47. Fred Nelson, Safe Reading and Computer Box Company, Linwood, Michigan, telephone conversaion with author, October 4, 1996.

48. Ed Hogan, telephone conversations with author, November 1991—October 1994.

49. James Dulley, "Electric Radiant Heaters are Safe and Efficient," *SMS Utility Bills Update*, No. 249, Cincinnati, March 7, 1992.

50. Wharton and Spring, *Spas, Hot Tubs*, 79.

51. Kenneth H. Cooper, M.D., *The Aerobic Program for Total Well-Being* (New York: Bantam Books, 1982) 13.

52. Saifer and Zellerbach, *Detox*, 72.

53. Kenneth Cooper, *The Aerobic Program*, 14–15.

54. *Ibid*. 112–115.

55. Environmental Health Center—Dallas, "Sauna Detoxification," photocopy, 2.

Bibliography

Amidon, Robert B. "Chemical Hazards in Law Enforcement," *Journal of California Law Enforcement* 18, 3 (Summer 1984) 27–30.

Ashford, Nicholas and Claudia Miller. *Chemical Exposures: Low Levels and High Stakes.* New York: Van Nostrand Reinhold, 1991.

Baker, Gordan P., M.D. "Porphyria and MCS Overlap Symptoms." *Our Toxic Times* 5, 8 (1994) 1–5.

Barron, Stephen R., M.D. *Survey of the Medical Impact on Environmentally Hypersensitive People of a Change in Habitat.* Ottawa: Canada Mortgage and Housing Corporation Publications, 1990.

Bower, John. *The Healthy House.* New York: Carol Publishing Group, 1993.

Brooks, Eugene C., IV. "Multiple Chemical Sensitivity Claims." Environmental and Toxic Tort Litigation Section, Association of Trial Lawyers of America, San Diego, Annual Convention (1990).

Browder, Sue, "Are You Allergic to the Modern World?" *Woman's Day* (April 1992) 56.

Callendar, Thomas J., Lisa Morrow, Kodanullar Subramanian, Dan Duhon, and Mona Ristovv, "Three-Dimensional Brain Metabolic Imaging in Patients with Toxic Encephalopathy," *Environmental Research* 60 (1993) 295–319.

Canada Mortgage and Housing Corporation. *Moisture and Air.* Ottawa: Canada Mortgage and Housing Corporation Publications, 1990.

Chen, Edwin. *PBB: An American Tragedy.* Englewood Cliffs, N.J.: Prentice-Hall, Inc., 1979.

Cohn, James R., M.S., and Edward A. Emmett, M.B., B.S., M.S., FRACP. "The Excretion of Trace Metals in Human Sweat." *Annals of Clinical and Laboratory Science* 8, 4 (1978) 270–274.

Cooper, Kenneth H., M.D. *The Aerobic Program for Total Well-Being.* New York: Bantam Books, 1982.

Crook, William G., M.D. *The Yeast Connection: A Medical Breakthrough.* Jackson, Tennessee: Professional Books, 1986.

Dadd, Debra L., *Non-Toxic, Natural & Earthwise.* Los Angeles: Jeremy P. Tarcher, Inc., 1990.

153

Davidoff, Linda L. "Multiple Chemical Sensitivities (MCS)," *The Amicus Journal* (Winter 1991) 14–23.

Drerup, Oliver, Chris Mattock, David Rousseau, and Virginia Salares. *Housing for the Environmentally Hypersensitive*. Ottawa: CMHC Publications, 1990.

Dulley, James. "Electric Radiant Heaters are Safe and Efficient," *SMS Utility Bills Update*, 249, Cincinnati, March 7, 1992.

Frisch, Tracy. *Multiple Chemical Sensitivity*. Albany: In the Workplace Taskforce, 1992.

Gibson, Mark, Gary Hoss, John Laseter, and William Rea., M.D. *Physician's Clinical Guide*. Dallas: Environmental Health Information Center, 1987.

Golos, Natalie, and Frances Golos Golbitz. *Coping with Your Allergies*. New York: Simon & Schuster, 1986.

Gorman, Carolyn P. *Less Toxic Living*. Dallas: Environmental Health Center, 1991.

Hileman, Bette. "Multiple Chemical Sensitivities." *Chemical & Engineering News*, 69 (July 1991) 26–41.

Heuser, Gunnar, M.D. "Diagnostic Markers in Clinical Immunotoxicology and Neurotoxicology." *Journal of Occupational Medicine and Toxicology* 1, 4 (1992).

Hubbard, L. Ron. *Clear Body: Clear Mind—The Effective Purification Program*. Los Angeles: Bridge Publications, Inc., 1990.

Human Ecology Action League. "Chemicals Can Affect Your Health." Atlanta, 1990.

Jacob, Stanley, M.D., and Clarice Ashworth Francone. *Structure and Function in Man*. Philadelphia: W. B. Saunders Co., 1965.

Jason, Leonard A., Ph.D., and Trina Davis. "M.C.S. Treatment Evaluation Survey of 305 Participants." DePaul University, undated.

Kilburn, K.H., M.D., R. Warsaw, and M. Shields, M.D. "Neurobehavioral Dysfunction in Firemen Exposed to Polychlorinated Biphenyls (PCBs): Possible Improvement after Detoxification." *Archives of Environmental Health* 44, 6 (1989) 345–349.

Kilburn, Kaye H., M.D. "Is the Human Nervous System Most Sensitive to Environmental Toxins?" *Archives of Environmental Health* 44, 6 (1989) 343–344.

Krohn, Jacqueline, M.D., Frances A. Taylor, M.A., and Erla Mae Larson, R.N. *The Whole Way to Allergy Relief and Prevention: A Doctor's Complete Guide to Treatment and Self Care*. Point Roberts, Washington: Hartley & Marks, Inc., 1991.

Lamielle, Mary. *Patients Held Hostage: A Collection of Articles on the Medical Controversy Surrounding MCS*. Voorhees, New Jersey: National Center for Environmental Health Strategies, 1989.

Marbella, Jean. "How We Sweat." *Baltimore Sun*, April 28, 1992.

Matthews, Bonnye L. *Chemical Sensitivity: A Guide to Coping with Hypersensitivity Syndrome, Sick Building Syndrome and Other Environmental Illnesses*. Jefferson, North Carolina: McFarland, 1992.

Meggs, William J., M.D., and Crawford H. Cleveland, Jr., M.D. "Rhinolaryngo-scopic Examination of Patients with the Multiple Chemical Sensitivity Syndrome." *Archives of Environmental Health* 48, 1 (1993) 14–18.

Metzger, Kathryn. "Glass Greenhouse Becomes Sauna." *The Human Ecologist* 49 (Summer 1991) 16.

Moll, Lucy. "Tell Me It's Not for Real." *Vegetarian Times* (October 1991) 56–65.

Morehouse, Laurence, and Augustus Miller, M.D. *Physiology of Exercise.* St. Louis: C.V. Mosby Co., 1967.

Rea, William J., M.D., FACS, FAAEM, "Environmental Illness." *The S.T.A.T.E.ment* (The S.T.A.T.E. Foundation, Orchard Park, New York) 1, 3 (Summer 1995) 1.

Regenstein, Lewis. *America the Poisoned.* Washington, D.C: Acropolis Books, Ltd., 1982.

Roehm, Dan Christian. "Effects of a Program of Sauna Baths and Megavitamins on Adipose DDE and PCBs and on Clearing of Symptoms of Agent Orange (Dioxin) Toxicity," *Clinical Research* 31, 2 (1983) 243A.

Rogers, Sherry A. *Tired or Toxic? A Blueprint for Health.* Syracuse: Prestige Publishing, 1990.

Root, David E., M.D., and Joan Anderson. "Reducing Toxic Body Burdens Advancing in Innovative Technique." *Occupational Health and Safety News Digest* 2, 4 (April 1986).

Root, David E., M.D., MPH, and Gerald T. Lionelli, B.S. "Excretion of a Lipophilic Toxicant Through the Sebaceous Glands: A Case Report." *Journal of Toxicology* 6, 1 (1987) 13–17.

Safran, Claire. "Schools That Make Kids Sick," *Good Housekeeping* (March 1992) 176–177, 254–259.

Saifer, Phyllis, M.D., and Merla Zellerbach. *Detox.* New York: Ballantine Books, 1984.

Schacker, Stephen A., M.D. "A Triune Brain Model of MCS Syndrome." *Our Toxic Times* 4, 7 (1993) 1–3.

Schnare, D. W., G. Denk, M. Shields, M.D., and S. Brunton. "Evaluation of a Detoxification Regimen for Fat Stored Xenobiotics." *Medical Hypotheses* 9 (1982) 265–282.

Schnare, David, Max Ben, and Megan Shields, M.D. "Body Burden Reductions of PCBs, PBBs, and Chlorinated Pesticides in Human Subjects." *Ambio* 13, 5–6 (1984) 378–380.

Small, Bruce, and Jim White. *Implications of Chemical Hypersensitivity for Housing Design.* Ottawa: CMHC Publications, 1990.

Swartz, Richard D., M.D. (Captain, MC, USA), and Frederick R. Sidell, M.D. "Effects of Heat and Exercise on the Elimination of Pralidoxime in Man." Clinical Investigation Section, Biomedical Laboratory, Edgewood Arsenal,

Maryland, paper presented in part at the Federation of American Societies for Experimental Biology Meeting, American Society for Pharmacology and Experimental Therapeutics Section, Atlantic City, N.J. (April 10, 1972).

Tretjak, Ziga, Shelley Beckman, Ana Tretjak, and Charles Gunnerson. "Occupational, Environmental, and Public Health in Semic: A Case Study of Polychlorinated Biphenyl (PCB) Pollution." Reprinted from *Post-Audits of Environmental Programs and Projects Proceedings*, Environmental Impact Analysis Research Council, ASCE, New Orleans (October 11, 1989) 57–72.

Warton, Susan, and Paul Spring. *Spas, Hot Tubs, and Home Saunas.* Menlo Park, California: Lane Publishing Co., 1989.

Wilson, Cynthia. *Chemical Exposure and Human Health: A Reference to 314 Chemicals, with a Guide to Symptoms and a Directory of Organizations.* Jefferson, North Carolina: McFarland, 1993.

Winter, Ruth. *A Consumer's Dictionary of Household, Yard and Office Chemicals.* New York: Crown Publishers, Inc., 1992.

Wolff, Mary S., Ph.D., Henry A. Anderson, M.D., and Irving J. Selikoff, M.D. "Human Tissue Burdens of Halogenated Aromatic Chemicals in Michigan." *Journal of the American Medical Association* 247, 15 (April 16, 1982) 2112–2116.

Wolff, Mary S., H. A. Anderson, K. D. Rosenman, and I. J. Selikoff. "Equilibrium of Polybrominated Biphenyl (PBB) Residues in Serum and Fat of Michigan Residents." *Bulletin of Environmental Contamination and Toxicology* 21, 6 (1979) 775–781.

Ziem, Grace E., M.D. "Multiple Chemical Sensitivity: Treatment and Follow-up with Avoidance and Control of Chemical Exposures." *Toxicology and Industrial Health*, 8 (1992) 73-86.

Ziem, Grace, M.D. "Diagnosing and Treating Chemically Injured People." *Pesticides and You* (Summer/Fall 1993) 8.

Index